OVERCOMING OVEREATING

A Behavior Oriented Program for Permanent Weight Control

Second Edition

Rick Guyton, Ph.D.
Jane Guyton, Ed.D.

GINN PRESS
160 Gould Street
Needham Heights, MA 02194

Printed in the United States of America

10 9 8 7 6 5 4 3 2 1

ISBN 0-536-58157-6
BA 2534

GINN PRESS

160 Gould Street/Needham Heights, MA 02194
Simon & Schuster Higher Education Publishing Group

Table of Contents

PREFACE

Overcoming Overeating is a comprehensive fat control program that has been designed to help people learn how to help themselves. The program includes a heavy emphasis on techniques that facilitate self understanding in personal eating habits and exercise regimens. It is our belief that "solutions to permanent fat control" are not achievable without a comprehensive approach to lifestyle change. This program represents our attempt to provide a behavior change system that is flexible enough to meet the needs of all types of personalities, yet structured enough to provide order and discipline to the individual who needs direction and leadership with a personal fat control plan. The "change system" is supplemented with the basic nutritional information and exercise information basic to self control and responsible decision making. The plan is designed to help participants lose 1-3 pounds weekly while developing new healthier nutritional habits and exercise regimens. The program may be attempted independently or this manual may serve as the guide for group oriented fat control programs.

PREFACE

Acknowledgments

The authors wish to thank many former students who have made suggestions for improvements; three special students who helped with this manuscript include Ms. Melody Taylor, Ms. Donna Reed, and Mr. Charles Mullins.

SELF UNDERSTANDING

NAME ______________________________ AGE __________

Answer **honestly:**

1. Do you like yourself at your present weight? ______________________________
2. What would you like to weigh? ______________________________
3. Do you consider yourself physically fit? ______________________________
4. What health problems do you have at this time that might be related to your being overfat?

____

____

____

5. How often do you weigh yourself? ______________________________
6. What are your three favorite foods? ______________________________

____

____

7. What are your three least favorite foods? ______________________________

____

____

8. If you were planning a menu, what would you include for:

   Breakfast: ______________________________

   Lunch (Dinner): ______________________________

   Dinner (Supper): ______________________________
9. What are your favorite snacks? ______________________________
10. Where do you eat most of your meals? (kitchen, TV room, etc.)

    ____
11. Do you skip meals in an effort to control your weight? ______________________________
12. Do you often snack between meals? ______________________________

13. When do you usually eat snacks? ____________________

14. Do you eat while you are doing other things? ____________________

15. What activities do you include with eating? (i.e., reading, watching TV, etc.)

____

____

16. Do you ever eat a whole package of snack foods? If so, what are your favorites?

____

____

17. Do you eat at regularly scheduled times of the day? ____________________
(Why or why not?) ____________________

18. Do you frequently eat when you are emotionally upset? ____________________

19. Do you generally eat family style with second helpings readily available? __________

20. Do you put your utensils down between bites of food? ____________________

21. Do you usually clean you plate? ____________________

22. Do you know the caloric values of the foods you consume? ____________________

23. Do you consume approximately the same number of calories each day? __________

24. Do you feel that not losing weight at a fast rate is a sign of failure? __________

25. Do you know the nutritional values of the foods you eat? ____________________

26. Are your foods prepared creatively and imaginatively? ____________________

27. Are you satisfied with your ability to discipline yourself when it comes to eating? ______

28. Are you mentally in control of the food you eat and the amount you eat? __________

29. What are your poorest eating habits? ____________________

____

30. Are you willing to adjust your present lifestyle and commit yourself to a comprehensive fatweight management program? ____________________

31. What or who are the strongest motivating factors in your life? ____________________

____

DO

Need RHR

Pre-Exercise Profile

Name ______________________________ Date ______________________________ Age __________

Body Weight __________________ Resting Heart Rate __________________
(1 minute pulse)

Percent Body Fat __________ Beginning Exercise Heart Rate __________________
(220 — present age x .60)

Body Fat Classification ______________________

Do you have any known physical handicaps? ______________________________

____

____

What are your major recreational interests? ______________________________

____

____

What kind of recreational facilities are most available to you each day? __________

____

____

What is your best time(s) of day to exercise? ______________________________

____

Do you belong to a fitness center, spa, country club, health club, or special organization that offers exercise opportunity?

Yes ______ No ______ Identify ______________________________

	Activity	Comments
________	Jogging	______________________________
________	Swimming	______________________________
________	Walking	______________________________
________	Cycling	______________________________
________	Tennis	______________________________
________	Racquetball	______________________________
________	Dancing	______________________________
________	Rebounding	______________________________

How Many Calories Do I Need Each Day?

The number of calories needed to maintain ideal weight is directly proportional to your daily
exercise habits. Identify your present exercise level utilizing the following scale:

12 No exercise other than sitting or lying down.

13 No regular exercise, very sedentary.

14 Daily walking, but not anything strenuous, or planned.

15 Active every day with a planned program of jogging, rebounding, swimming, cycling or some form of aerobic exercises.

16 Daily aerobic exercise for periods exceeding 90 minutes of intense activity.

Enter the number that best describes your daily exercise habits here _______ , and multiply it time your ideal weight.

If you are 13 with no regular exercise and your ideal weight is 120, it would be calculated as follows:

13 x 120 = 1,560 each day

My daily caloric needs to maintain my ideal weight is __________

To reach my goal of __________ pounds, I will decrease my caloric consumption to __________ calories each day.

This total of course is only an approximation of your daily caloric needs. If you desire to lose weight, you should decrease your daily consumption by 100+ calories and add daily aerobic exercise to help burn the additional stored calories contributing to your overweight condition.

Once you have determined how many calories you need each day, memorize that number and limit your daily caloric intake to that amount. If you will initiate a daily exercise program of 30 to 40 minutes and monitor your caloric intake, you should be able to balance your caloric intake/exercise expenditure. The best solution to permanent weight management is sensible eating and an active lifestyle. Use this manual as a resource, to expand your knowledge of the important relationship between exercise and nutrition.

THE RECORD KEEPING COMPONEN

This weight control program lasts eight weeks. Each week you will keep records to help you understand more about your present eating and exercise behaviors. You will find out which behaviors to reinforce, which ones to eliminate, and which ones to modify. The program is based on the fact that changing eating habits combined with moderate exercise, is the most effective, safe, and permanent means of weight control.

On the following page you will see an eating and exercise diary, an important record keeping component of the program. Completing the eating and exercise diary each day is essential if your program is to be successful. Note that the eating and exercise diary consists of the following parts.

UNDERSTANDING THE DAILY FOOD AND EXERCISE DIARY

I. Strategy for the Week

Developing weekly strategies to modify your eating behavior helps you reach your goal of permanent weight loss more readily. You should chose one of your problem areas listed in your Problem Eating Inventory for the Week (p. 8) and decide on a strategy to address this problem. List the strategy in the space provided at the top of the diary.

II. Daily Caloric Quota Reminder

You have already figured your (daily caloric quota) by multiplying your ideal weight times your degree of activity and subtracting 100 calories (p. 4). At the beginning of each day, write down your daily caloric quota in the right-hand corner of the eating diary in the indicated square. Having a daily caloric quota serves as a goal and helps you more accurately plan your daily food intake.

III. Time of Eating

It is important to indicate when you eat. Writing down the time you eat will enable you to identify and modify your pattern of food consumption throughout the day. Eventually you will want to eat more of your food earlier in the day when you are more active and reduce late night meals and snacking.

IV. Food Quality and Calories

Write down all the food you eat and estimate as closely as possible the quantity and calories of each item. Use the calorie counter included in the back of the manual. Listing everything you eat and the calories helps you to see the total amount of food you eat each day and the number of calories you consume over your daily caloric quota.

V. Meal or Snack

Indicate if the food eaten is a Meal (M) or Snack (S). The objective of this component is for you to become aware of and modify the number of times you eat and the number of times you snack each day.

VI. **Where Consumed**

Write down where you eat your meal or snack (i.e., kitchen table, car, in front of the T.V.). From this information you can become aware of how your environment may stimulate you to overeat. Eventually you will want to limit most of your eating to only one eating place.

VII. **Feelings Before Eating**

Indicate how you feel immediately before you eat (i.e., happy, rushed, frustrated). This helps you know yourself and helps you become aware of the events and the emotions which cause you to overeat.

Below the eating diary are additional questions you need to ask yourself each day.

1. Did you eat something from each of the Four Basic Food Groups? It is important that you not only reduce your caloric intake but that you eat a variety of good healthy foods each day. To ensure that you are eating the food necessary for your body's daily needs, you should make your food selection from each of the Four Basic Food Groups. The 4-2-2-4 Formula is recommended for adults. Each day plan for:

   4 servings — bread and cereal (small portions)
   2 servings — milk and milk products (low fat)
   2 servings — meat (fish and poultry recommended)
   4 servings — vegetables and fruits (dark green and yellow vegetables, 1 citrus fruit daily)

2. Did you consume most of your food before 2:00 p.m.?
   It is best to eat most of your food during the day when you are most active rather than in the evening when you are less active. Eating food earlier in the day will give you the necessary source of energy for your daily activities and be less readily turned to fat.

3. Did you eat all of your food at the same designated place?
   Your environment may stimulate you to overeat. By reducing your eating to only one place you can eliminate unnecessary snacking and enjoy more planned meals instead.

4. Did you stay within ± 200 caloric quota?
   The ±200 calories around your caloric quota give you an approximate range for your caloric intake. As long as your stay within this range, you will find that you can lose weight comfortably and safely.

5. Did you have a planned exercise time for the day?
   Plan your daily schedule to include at least 30 minutes of continuous aerobic exercise. Planning your exercise session cannot be overemphasized. If you don't plan it, other activities may take priority.

   Following each exercise session, indicate the type of aerobic activity, how long you exercised, and your approximate target heart rate during exercise.

Sample

Daily Food and Exercise Diary

(for self record keeping)

Day of Week *Tuesday*

Strategy for the Week *Switch to diet colas*

Daily Caloric Quota Reminder	Daily Fat Gram Budget
1400	*47*

Time	Food	Quantity	Meal or Snack	Where Consumed	Feelings Before Eating	Calories	Fat in Grams
6:00 a.m.	Raisin Bran	1 bowl	M	Kitchen	Sleepy	110	1
	Skim milk	1 cup	M	Kitchen	Sleepy	90	0
10:00 a.m.	Quarter pounder with cheese	1	M	McDonald's	Starving	524	30
	French fries	1 small	M	McDonald's	Starving	220	12
	Diet Coke	Large	M	McDonald's	Starving	0	0
2:00 p.m	Apple	1 med.	S	T.V. Lounge	Bored	80	0
	Diet Coke	Large	S	Michele's room	Bored	0	0
6:00 p.m.	Green beans	1 cup	M	Dining room	Hungry	44	0
	Round steak (Fat trimmed)	3 oz.	M	Dining room	Hungry	220	8
	Roll	1 med.	M	Dining room	Hungry	100	2
						1388	

1. Did you eat something from each of the 4 basic food groups? Yes / No
   Milk ___ Meat ___ Fruit & Vegetable ___ Grains ___
2. Did you consume most of your food before 2:00 p.m.? Yes / No
3. Did you eat all of your food at the same designated place? Yes / No
4. Did you stay ± 200 calories of your caloric quota? Yes / No
5. Did you stay ± 5 grams of your fat gram budget? Yes / No
6. Did you have a planned exercise time for the day? Yes / No

If yes: Type ______________________

Duration ______________________

Approximate Heart Rate ______________________

Sample

Problem Inventory for the Week

Each day check those items that you perceive as problems that make you want to overeat. At the end of the week, total the number of days during the week each item was a problem.	M	T	W	TH	F	S	SU	TOTAL
1. Snacks	✓	✓	✓	✓	✓	✓	✓	7
2. High Fat	✓	✓			✓			3
3. Sugar								
4. Fast Food Establishments	✓	✓		✓				3
5. Troublesome Foods	✓	✓			✓	✓		4
6. Eat Until Full or Overfull	✓	✓						2
7. Candy								
8. Coffee								
9. Non-diet Cola Drinks	✓	✓				✓		3
10. Alcohol								
11. Doughnuts								
12. Salad Dressings	✓							1
13. Lack of Home Support								
14. Restaurants	✓						✓	2
15. Big Meals								
16. Unaware of Food Consumption	✓	✓	✓	✓		✓		5
17. Too Much Red Meat								
18. Craving Certain Food								
19. Social Events	✓					✓		2
20. Desserts								
21. No Exercise	✓	✓	✓					3
22. Lack of Friendly Support								
23. Lack of Motivation	✓	✓	✓					3

Now rank the three problems that you feel are contributing most to your tendency to overeat.

1. *snacks*
2. *unaware of food consumption*
3. *troublesome foods*

SAMPLE

PERSONAL ACTION PLAN

I. Problem: Snacking

II. Strategies for the Problem

(1) Plan for snacks, eat low calorie snacks instead

(2) Remove myself from the temptation to snack

(3) Write a list of alternatives to eating

(4) Write a contract with my roommate

III. Best Strategy for the Problem

Plan for snacks—buy & eat low calorie snacks instead of high calorie snacks

IV. Weekly Reward

I will reward myself with a new shirt if I am responsible and consistent with this week's strategy.

V. Statement of Commitment

For this wek, I will buy fresh apples, bananas, oranges, & carrots to eat instead of high calorie snacks

Suggested Weights for Adults

Height[1]	Weight in Pounds[2]	
	19 to 34 years	36 years and over
5'0"	[3]97-128	108-138
5'1"	101-132	111-143
5'2"	104-137	115-148
5'3"	107-141	119-152
5'4"	111-146	122-157
5'5"	114-150	126-162
5'6"	118-155	130-167
5'7"	121-160	134-172
5'8"	125-164	138-178
5'9"	129-169	142-183
5'10"	132-174	146-188
5'11"	136-179	151-194
6'0"	140-184	155-199
6'1"	144-189	159-205
6'2"	148-195	164-210
6'3"	152-200	168-216
6'4"	156-205	173-222
6'5"	160-211	177-228
6'6"	164-216	182-234

[1]Without shoes.

[2]Without clothes.

[3]The higher weights in the ranges generally apply to men, who tend to have more muscle and bone; the lower weights more often apply to women, who have less muscle and bone.

Source: Derived from National Research Council.

The Record Keeping Plan for Overcoming Overeating

EIGHT-WEEK BEHAVIORAL CHANGE CONTRACT

Before beginning your behavioral change program, you should get the support of a friend or relative to help you lose weight. The behavioral change contract which you and your friend or relative will sign should consist of both short-term and long-term weight loss goals with the weight loss not exceeding two pounds each week. As part of the contract, you should establish an adequate reward system to help motivate you to complete the eight-week program. A monetary reward is usually ideal, such as setting aside fifty dollars to spend as you wish, if you successfully complete the program. It is advisable to establish a weekly reward system as well for completing the necessary forms and following the prescribed program. Under no circumstances should food or alcohol be rewards. Fill out the contract below and sign as indicated.

EIGHT WEEK BEHAVIORAL CHANGE CONTRACT

GOAL

Through utilization of lifestyle modification strategies presented in this program,

I ____ (name)

agree to attempt to reduce my weight during the next three months.

OBJECTIVES

A. In 8 weeks, I propose to weigh _____ lbs. (Do not set a goal exceeding two pounds per week.)

A. In 3 months, I propose to weigh _____ lbs. (Do not set a goal exceeding two pounds per week.)

REWARDS

If I achieve my goals, my reward(s) will be

____

____

____

____

______________________________	______________________________
Signature (1st person)	Signature (2nd person)

DAILY FOOD AND EXERCISE DIARY

Day of Week ______________________

Strategy for the Week ______________________

Daily Caloric Quota Reminder

Daily Fat Gram Budget

Time	Food	Quantity	Meal or Snack	Where Consumed	Feelings Before Eating	Calories	Fat in Grams

1. Did you eat something from each of the 4 basic food groups? **Yes / No**
   Milk ___ Meat ___ Fruit & Vegetable ___ Grains ___
2. Did you consume most of your food before 2:00 p.m.? **Yes / No**
3. Did you eat all of your food at the same designated place? **Yes / No**
4. Did you stay ± 200 calories of your caloric quota? **Yes / No**
5. Did you stay ± 5 grams of your fat gram budget? **Yes / No**
6. Did you have a planned exercise time for the day? **Yes / No**

   If yes: Type ______________________

   Duration ______________________

   Approximate Heart Rate ______________________

WEEK 1

DAILY FOOD AND EXERCISE DIARY

Day of Week ______________________________

Strategy for the Week ______________________

Daily Caloric Quota Reminder [ ]

Daily Fat Gram Budget [ ]

Time	Food	Quantity	Meal or Snack	Where Consumed	Feelings Before Eating	Calories	Fat in Grams

1. Did you eat something from each of the 4 basic food groups? **Yes / No**
   Milk ___ Meat ___ Fruit & Vegetable ___ Grains ___
2. Did you consume most of your food before 2:00 p.m.? **Yes / No**
3. Did you eat all of your food at the same designated place? **Yes / No**
4. Did you stay ± 200 calories of your caloric quota? **Yes / No**
5. Did you stay ± 5 grams of your fat gram budget? **Yes / No**
6. Did you have a planned exercise time for the day? **Yes / No**

If yes: Type ______________________________

Duration ______________________________

Approximate Heart Rate ______________________

WEEK 1

DAILY FOOD AND EXERCISE DIARY

Day of Week ______________________

Strategy for the Week ______________________

Daily Caloric Quota Reminder [ ]

Daily Fat Gram Budget [ ]

Time	Food	Quantity	Meal or Snack	Where Consumed	Feelings Before Eating	Calories	Fat in Grams

1. Did you eat something from each of the 4 basic food groups? **Yes / No**
   Milk ___ Meat ___ Fruit & Vegetable ___ Grains ___
2. Did you consume most of your food before 2:00 p.m.? **Yes / No**
3. Did you eat all of your food at the same designated place? **Yes / No**
4. Did you stay ± 200 calories of your caloric quota? **Yes / No**
5. Did you stay ± 5 grams of your fat gram budget? **Yes / No**
6. Did you have a planned exercise time for the day? **Yes / No**

If yes: Type ______________________

Duration ______________________

Approximate Heart Rate ______________________

WEEK 1

DAILY FOOD AND EXERCISE DIARY

Day of Week ____________________

Strategy for the Week ____________________

Daily Caloric Quota Reminder	Daily Fat Gram Budget

Time	Food	Quantity	Meal or Snack	Where Consumed	Feelings Before Eating	Calories	Fat in Grams

1. Did you eat something from each of the 4 basic food groups? **Yes / No**
   Milk ___ Meat ___ Fruit & Vegetable ___ Grains ___
2. Did you consume most of your food before 2:00 p.m.? **Yes / No**
3. Did you eat all of your food at the same designated place? **Yes / No**
4. Did you stay ± 200 calories of your caloric quota? **Yes / No**
5. Did you stay ± 5 grams of your fat gram budget? **Yes / No**
6. Did you have a planned exercise time for the day? **Yes / No**

   If yes: Type ____________________

   Duration ____________________

   Approximate Heart Rate ____________________

WEEK 1

DAILY FOOD AND EXERCISE DIARY

Day of Week ____________________

Strategy for the Week ____________________

Daily Caloric Quota Reminder [ ]

Daily Fat Gram Budget [ ]

Time	Food	Quantity	Meal or Snack	Where Consumed	Feelings Before Eating	Calories	Fat in Grams

1. Did you eat something from each of the 4 basic food groups? **Yes / No**
   Milk ___ Meat ___ Fruit & Vegetable ___ Grains ___
2. Did you consume most of your food before 2:00 p.m.? **Yes / No**
3. Did you eat all of your food at the same designated place? **Yes / No**
4. Did you stay ± 200 calories of your caloric quota? **Yes / No**
5. Did you stay ± 5 grams of your fat gram budget? **Yes / No**
6. Did you have a planned exercise time for the day? **Yes / No**

   If yes: Type ____________________

   Duration ____________________

   Approximate Heart Rate ____________________

Week 1

Daily Food and Exercise Diary

Day of Week ______________________

Strategy for the Week ______________________

Daily Caloric Quota Reminder	Daily Fat Gram Budget

Time	Food	Quantity	Meal or Snack	Where Consumed	Feelings Before Eating	Calories	Fat in Grams

1. Did you eat something from each of the 4 basic food groups? **Yes / No**
   Milk ___ Meat ___ Fruit & Vegetable ___ Grains ___
2. Did you consume most of your food before 2:00 p.m.? **Yes / No**
3. Did you eat all of your food at the same designated place? **Yes / No**
4. Did you stay ± 200 calories of your caloric quota? **Yes / No**
5. Did you stay ± 5 grams of your fat gram budget? **Yes / No**
6. Did you have a planned exercise time for the day? **Yes / No**

   If yes: Type ______________________

   Duration ______________________

   Approximate Heart Rate ______________________

WEEK 1

DAILY FOOD AND EXERCISE DIARY

Day of Week ______________________________

Strategy for the Week ______________________

Daily Caloric Quota Reminder [ ]

Daily Fat Gram Budget [ ]

Time	Food	Quantity	Meal or Snack	Where Consumed	Feelings Before Eating	Calories	Fat in Grams

1. Did you eat something from each of the 4 basic food groups? **Yes / No**
   Milk ___ Meat ___ Fruit & Vegetable ___ Grains ___
2. Did you consume most of your food before 2:00 p.m.? **Yes / No**
3. Did you eat all of your food at the same designated place? **Yes / No**
4. Did you stay ± 200 calories of your caloric quota? **Yes / No**
5. Did you stay ± 5 grams of your fat gram budget? **Yes / No**
6. Did you have a planned exercise time for the day? **Yes / No**

If yes: Type ______________________________

Duration ______________________________

Approximate Heart Rate ______________________

Week 1

Problem Inventory for the Week

Each day check those items that you perceive as problems that make you want to overeat. At the end of the week, total the number of days during the week each item was a problem.	M	T	W	TH	F	S	SU	TOTAL
1. Snacks								
2. High Fat								
3. Sugar								
4. Fast Food Establishments								
5. Troublesome Foods								
6. Eat Until Full or Overfull								
7. Candy								
8. Coffee								
9. Non-diet Cola Drinks								
10. Alcohol								
11. Doughnuts								
12. Salad Dressings								
13. Lack of Home Support								
14. Restaurants								
15. Big Meals								
16. Unaware of Food Consumption								
17. Too Much Red Meat								
18. Craving Certain Food								
19. Social Events								
20. Desserts								
21. No Exercise								
22. Lack of Friendly Support								
23. Lack of Motivation								

Now rank the three problems that you feel are contributing most to your tendency to overeat.

1. ______________________________
2. ______________________________
3. ______________________________

YOUR 8-STEP PERSONAL ACTION PLAN

Each week you will design your own individual Personal Action Plan. This plan, designed by you, consists of weight loss goals and strategies for the next week.

1. Weigh yourself and plot your weight on the Weight Loss Profile Sheet (p. 158).
2. Review your Eating and Exercise Diary and Problem Inventory for the week. Identify any problem eating behaviors that need to be corrected.
3. Select one problem eating behavior and describe it in this week's Personal Action Plan (as shown on the following page).
4. Write down several strategies that you could use to alter this selected problem eating behavior. From these strategies, select a best strategy as a solution and include this strategy in next week's Eating and Exercise Diary. Write the strategy in the space provided at the top of next week's Eating and Exercise Diary.
5. Consult with your partner in planning your complete program for the next week.
6. Plan your daily meal and exercise schedules for next week.
7. Indicate your commitment to the weekly Plan of Action by writing a personal statement of commitment.
8. Develop appropriate rewards for successful completion of the selected strategy.

Personal Action Plan

I. **Problem:** ______________________________

II. **Strategies for the Problem**

III. **Best Strategy for the Problem**

IV. **Weekly Reward**

V. **Statement of Commitment**

Self-Understanding Exercises

Alternative Activities

____________	Taking a walk	____________	Running errands
____________	Talking with a friend	____________	Brushing your teeth
____________	Reading	____________	Swimming
____________	Studying	____________	Playing card games
____________	Taking a shower	____________	Jogging
____________	Cooking	____________	Riding a bicycle
____________	Playing tennis	____________	Calling a friend or relative
____________	Playing golf	____________	Calling a friend or relative
____________	Eating low cal snacks	____________	Knitting, crocheting, or embroidering
____________	Drinking water	____________	Writing a letter to a friend or relative
____________	Going for a drive	____________	Ironing

This week, the specific activities I will use to control my weight are:

Recreational Activities	**Work Activities**
______________________________	______________________________
______________________________	______________________________
______________________________	______________________________

What daily situations are most likely to initiate your need to use the activities listed above?

____

____

____

____

WEEK 2

DAILY FOOD AND EXERCISE DIARY

Day of Week ______________________________

Strategy for the Week ______________________

Daily Caloric Quota Reminder	**Daily Fat Gram Budget**

Time	**Food**	**Quantity**	**Meal or Snack**	**Where Consumed**	**Feelings Before Eating**	**Calories**	**Fat in Grams**

1. Did you eat something from each of the 4 basic food groups? **Yes / No**
   Milk ___ Meat ___ Fruit & Vegetable ___ Grains ___
2. Did you consume most of your food before 2:00 p.m.? **Yes / No**
3. Did you eat all of your food at the same designated place? **Yes / No**
4. Did you stay ± 200 calories of your caloric quota? **Yes / No**
5. Did you stay ± 5 grams of your fat gram budget? **Yes / No**
6. Did you have a planned exercise time for the day? **Yes / No**

   If yes: Type ______________________________

   Duration ______________________________

   Approximate Heart Rate ______________________

WEEK 2

DAILY FOOD AND EXERCISE DIARY

Day of Week ____________________

Strategy for the Week ____________________

Daily Caloric Quota Reminder	Daily Fat Gram Budget

Time	Food	Quantity	Meal or Snack	Where Consumed	Feelings Before Eating	Calories	Fat in Grams

1. Did you eat something from each of the 4 basic food groups? **Yes / No**

   Milk ___ Meat ___ Fruit & Vegetable ___ Grains ___
2. Did you consume most of your food before 2:00 p.m.? **Yes / No**
3. Did you eat all of your food at the same designated place? **Yes / No**
4. Did you stay ± 200 calories of your caloric quota? **Yes / No**
5. Did you stay ± 5 grams of your fat gram budget? **Yes / No**
6. Did you have a planned exercise time for the day? **Yes / No**

   If yes: Type ____________________

   Duration ____________________

   Approximate Heart Rate ____________________

Week 2

Daily Food and Exercise Diary

Day of Week ________________________

Strategy for the Week ________________________

Daily Caloric Quota Reminder	Daily Fat Gram Budget

Time	Food	Quantity	Meal or Snack	Where Consumed	Feelings Before Eating	Calories	Fat in Grams

1. Did you eat something from each of the 4 basic food groups? **Yes / No**
   Milk ___ Meat ___ Fruit & Vegetable ___ Grains ___
2. Did you consume most of your food before 2:00 p.m.? **Yes / No**
3. Did you eat all of your food at the same designated place? **Yes / No**
4. Did you stay ± 200 calories of your caloric quota? **Yes / No**
5. Did you stay ± 5 grams of your fat gram budget? **Yes / No**
6. Did you have a planned exercise time for the day? **Yes / No**

   If yes: Type ________________________

   Duration ________________________

   Approximate Heart Rate ____________________

WEEK 2

DAILY FOOD AND EXERCISE DIARY

Day of Week ______________________________

Strategy for the Week ______________________

Daily Caloric Quota Reminder	Daily Fat Gram Budget

Time	Food	Quantity	Meal or Snack	Where Consumed	Feelings Before Eating	Calories	Fat in Grams

1. Did you eat something from each of the 4 basic food groups? **Yes / No**
   Milk ___ Meat ___ Fruit & Vegetable ___ Grains ___
2. Did you consume most of your food before 2:00 p.m.? **Yes / No**
3. Did you eat all of your food at the same designated place? **Yes / No**
4. Did you stay $\pm$ 200 calories of your caloric quota? **Yes / No**
5. Did you stay $\pm$ 5 grams of your fat gram budget? **Yes / No**
6. Did you have a planned exercise time for the day? **Yes / No**

   If yes: Type ______________________________

   Duration ______________________________

   Approximate Heart Rate ______________________

Week 2

Daily Food and Exercise Diary

Day of Week ______________________________

Strategy for the Week ______________________

Daily Caloric Quota Reminder

Daily Fat Gram Budget

Time	Food	Quantity	Meal or Snack	Where Consumed	Feelings Before Eating	Calories	Fat in Grams

1. Did you eat something from each of the 4 basic food groups? **Yes / No**
   Milk ___ Meat ___ Fruit & Vegetable ___ Grains ___
2. Did you consume most of your food before 2:00 p.m.? **Yes / No**
3. Did you eat all of your food at the same designated place? **Yes / No**
4. Did you stay $\pm$ 200 calories of your caloric quota? **Yes / No**
5. Did you stay $\pm$ 5 grams of your fat gram budget? **Yes / No**
6. Did you have a planned exercise time for the day? **Yes / No**

If yes: Type ______________________________

Duration ______________________________

Approximate Heart Rate ______________________

WEEK 2

DAILY FOOD AND EXERCISE DIARY

Day of Week ______________________

Strategy for the Week ______________________

Daily Caloric Quota Reminder	Daily Fat Gram Budget

Time	Food	Quantity	Meal or Snack	Where Consumed	Feelings Before Eating	Calories	Fat in Grams

1. Did you eat something from each of the 4 basic food groups? **Yes / No**
   Milk ___ Meat ___ Fruit & Vegetable ___ Grains ___
2. Did you consume most of your food before 2:00 p.m.? **Yes / No**
3. Did you eat all of your food at the same designated place? **Yes / No**
4. Did you stay ± 200 calories of your caloric quota? **Yes / No**
5. Did you stay ± 5 grams of your fat gram budget? **Yes / No**
6. Did you have a planned exercise time for the day? **Yes / No**

   If yes: Type ______________________

   Duration ______________________

   Approximate Heart Rate ______________________

WEEK 2

DAILY FOOD AND EXERCISE DIARY

Day of Week ______________________

Strategy for the Week ______________________

Daily Caloric Quota Reminder	Daily Fat Gram Budget

Time	Food	Quantity	Meal or Snack	Where Consumed	Feelings Before Eating	Calories	Fat in Grams

1. Did you eat something from each of the 4 basic food groups? **Yes / No**
   Milk ___ Meat ___ Fruit & Vegetable ___ Grains ___
2. Did you consume most of your food before 2:00 p.m.? **Yes / No**
3. Did you eat all of your food at the same designated place? **Yes / No**
4. Did you stay ± 200 calories of your caloric quota? **Yes / No**
5. Did you stay ± 5 grams of your fat gram budget? **Yes / No**
6. Did you have a planned exercise time for the day? **Yes / No**

If yes: Type ______________________

Duration ______________________

Approximate Heart Rate ______________________

WEEK 2

PROBLEM INVENTORY FOR THE WEEK

Each day check those items that you perceive as problems that make you want to overeat. At the end of the week, total the number of days during the week each item was a problem.

	M	T	W	T	F	S	S	TOTAL
1. Snacks								
2. High Fat								
3. Sugar								
4. Fast Food Establishments								
5. Troublesome Foods								
6. Eat Until Full or Overfull								
7. Candy								
8. Coffee								
9. Non-diet Cola Drinks								
10. Alcohol								
11. Doughnuts								
12. Salad Dressings								
13. Lack of Home Support								
14. Restaurants								
15. Big Meals								
16. Unaware of Food Consumption								
17. Too Much Red Meat								
18. Craving Certain Food								
19. Social Events								
20. Desserts								
21. No Exercise								
22. Lack of Friendly Support								
23. Lack of Motivation								

Now rank the three problems that you feel are contributing most to your tendency to overeat.

1. ______________________________

2. ______________________________

3. ______________________________

YOUR 8-STEP PERSONAL ACTION PLAN

Each week you will design your own individual Personal Action Plan. This plan, designed by you, consists of weight loss goals and strategies for the next week.

1. Weigh yourself and plot your weight on the Weight Loss Profile Sheet (p. 158).
2. Review your Eating and Exercise Diary and Problem Inventory for the week. Identify any problem eating behaviors that need to be corrected.
3. Select one problem eating behavior and describe it in this week's Personal Action Plan (as shown on the following page).
4. Write down several strategies that you could use to alter this selected problem eating behavior. From these strategies, select a best strategy as a solution and include this strategy in next week's Eating and Exercise Diary. Write the strategy in the space provided at the top of next week's Eating and Exercise Diary.
5. Consult with your partner in planning your complete program for the next week.
6. Plan your daily meal and exercise schedules for next week.
7. Indicate your commitment to the weekly Plan of Action by writing a personal statement of commitment.
8. Develop appropriate rewards for successful completion of the selected strategy.

Personal Action Plan

I. **Problem:** ______________________________

II. **Strategies for the Problem**

III. **Best Strategy for the Problem**

IV. **Weekly Reward**

V. **Statement of Commitment**

Self-Understanding Exercises

Knowing Why You Eat

It is important to know why you eat. Do you . . .

- **Eat to Unwind**—many people eat immediately when they come home from work.
- **Eat Out of Boredom**—because you're away from your family, live alone, or don't have projects to do.
- **Eat Out of Tradition**—3 large meals a day is a cultural habit; not an established need.
- **Eat Out of Frustration**—a common pitfall for people who feel stressed, impatient, or angry.
- **Eat to be Entertained**—food is a readily available form of entertainment.
- **Eat Because Food Is Available**—food is easy to get with prepacked foods, microwaves, and drive throughs.
- **Eat Socially**—not really hungry but want to feel included.
- **Eat Because You Deserve it**—many people eat as a reward to make them feel better after a hard day.

Understanding yourself and why you eat is a helpful step toward effective weight control. Consider food as fuel to live rather than as a source of pleasure. Ask yourself, do you need this food or do you just want it. Think in terms of eating to live rather than living to eat.

WEEK 3

DAILY FOOD AND EXERCISE DIARY

Day of Week ______________________

Strategy for the Week ______________________

Daily Caloric Quota Reminder	Daily Fat Gram Budget

Time	Food	Quantity	Meal or Snack	Where Consumed	Feelings Before Eating	Calories	Fat in Grams

1. Did you eat something from each of the 4 basic food groups? **Yes / No**
   Milk ___ Meat ___ Fruit & Vegetable ___ Grains ___
2. Did you consume most of your food before 2:00 p.m.? **Yes / No**
3. Did you eat all of your food at the same designated place? **Yes / No**
4. Did you stay ± 200 calories of your caloric quota? **Yes / No**
5. Did you stay ± 5 grams of your fat gram budget? **Yes / No**
6. Did you have a planned exercise time for the day? **Yes / No**

   If yes: Type ______________________

   Duration ______________________

   Approximate Heart Rate ______________________

WEEK 3

DAILY FOOD AND EXERCISE DIARY

Day of Week ______________________

Strategy for the Week ________________

Daily Caloric Quota Reminder	Daily Fat Gram Budget

Time	Food	Quantity	Meal or Snack	Where Consumed	Feelings Before Eating	Calories	Fat In Grams

1. Did you eat something from each of the 4 basic food groups? **Yes / No**
   Milk ___ Meat ___ Fruit & Vegetable ___ Grains ___
2. Did you consume most of your food before 2:00 p.m.? **Yes / No**
3. Did you eat all of your food at the same designated place? **Yes / No**
4. Did you stay ± 200 calories of your caloric quota? **Yes / No**
5. Did you stay ± 5 grams of your fat gram budget? **Yes / No**
6. Did you have a planned exercise time for the day? **Yes / No**

If yes: Type ______________________

Duration ______________________

Approximate Heart Rate ______________________

WEEK 3

DAILY FOOD AND EXERCISE DIARY

Day of Week ______________________________

Strategy for the Week ______________________

Daily Caloric Quota Reminder [ ]

Daily Fat Gram Budget [ ]

Time	Food	Quantity	Meal or Snack	Where Consumed	Feelings Before Eating	Calories	Fat in Grams

1. Did you eat something from each of the 4 basic food groups? **Yes / No**
   Milk ___ Meat ___ Fruit & Vegetable ___ Grains ___
2. Did you consume most of your food before 2:00 p.m.? **Yes / No**
3. Did you eat all of your food at the same designated place? **Yes / No**
4. Did you stay ± 200 calories of your caloric quota? **Yes / No**
5. Did you stay ± 5 grams of your fat gram budget? **Yes / No**
6. Did you have a planned exercise time for the day? **Yes / No**

   If yes: Type ______________________________

   Duration ______________________________

   Approximate Heart Rate ____________________

WEEK 3

DAILY FOOD AND EXERCISE DIARY

Day of Week ______________________________

Strategy for the Week ______________________

Daily Caloric Quota Reminder	Daily Fat Gram Budget

Time	Food	Quantity	Meal or Snack	Where Consumed	Feelings Before Eating	Calories	Fat in Grams

1. Did you eat something from each of the 4 basic food groups? **Yes / No**
   Milk ___ Meat ___ Fruit & Vegetable ___ Grains ___
2. Did you consume most of your food before 2:00 p.m.? **Yes / No**
3. Did you eat all of your food at the same designated place? **Yes / No**
4. Did you stay ± 200 calories of your caloric quota? **Yes / No**
5. Did you stay ± 5 grams of your fat gram budget? **Yes / No**
6. Did you have a planned exercise time for the day? **Yes / No**

   If yes: Type ______________________________

   Duration ______________________________

   Approximate Heart Rate ______________________

WEEK 3

DAILY FOOD AND EXERCISE DIARY

Day of Week ______________________________

Strategy for the Week ______________________

Daily Caloric Quota Reminder	Daily Fat Gram Budget

Time	Food	Quantity	Meal or Snack	Where Consumed	Feelings Before Eating	Calories	Fat in Grams

1. Did you eat something from each of the 4 basic food groups? **Yes / No**
   Milk ___ Meat ___ Fruit & Vegetable ___ Grains ___
2. Did you consume most of your food before 2:00 p.m.? **Yes / No**
3. Did you eat all of your food at the same designated place? **Yes / No**
4. Did you stay ± 200 calories of your caloric quota? **Yes / No**
5. Did you stay ± 5 grams of your fat gram budget? **Yes / No**
6. Did you have a planned exercise time for the day? **Yes / No**

   If yes: Type ______________________________

   Duration ______________________________

   Approximate Heart Rate ______________________

WEEK 3

DAILY FOOD AND EXERCISE DIARY

Day of Week ______________________________

Strategy for the Week ______________________

Daily Caloric Quota Reminder [ ]

Daily Fat Gram Budget [ ]

Time	Food	Quantity	Meal or Snack	Where Consumed	Feelings Before Eating	Calories	Fat in Grams

1. Did you eat something from each of the 4 basic food groups? **Yes / No**
   Milk ___ Meat ___ Fruit & Vegetable ___ Grains ___
2. Did you consume most of your food before 2:00 p.m.? **Yes / No**
3. Did you eat all of your food at the same designated place? **Yes / No**
4. Did you stay ± 200 calories of your caloric quota? **Yes / No**
5. Did you stay ± 5 grams of your fat gram budget? **Yes / No**
6. Did you have a planned exercise time for the day? **Yes / No**

   If yes: Type ______________________________

   Duration ______________________________

   Approximate Heart Rate ______________________

WEEK 3

DAILY FOOD AND EXERCISE DIARY

Day of Week ________________________

Strategy for the Week ____________________

Daily Caloric Quota Reminder [ ]

Daily Fat Gram Budget [ ]

Time	Food	Quantity	Meal or Snack	Where Consumed	Feelings Before Eating	Calories	Fat in Grams

1. Did you eat something from each of the 4 basic food groups? **Yes / No**
   Milk ___ Meat ___ Fruit & Vegetable ___ Grains ___
2. Did you consume most of your food before 2:00 p.m.? **Yes / No**
3. Did you eat all of your food at the same designated place? **Yes / No**
4. Did you stay ± 200 calories of your caloric quota? **Yes / No**
5. Did you stay ± 5 grams of your fat gram budget? **Yes / No**
6. Did you have a planned exercise time for the day? **Yes / No**

   If yes: Type ____________________________

   Duration ____________________________

   Approximate Heart Rate ____________________

Week 3

Problem Inventory for the Week

Each day check those items that you perceive as problems that make you want to overeat. At the end of the week, total the number of days during the week each item was a problem.	M	T	W	T	F	S	S	TOTAL
1. Snacks								
2. High Fat								
3. Sugar								
4. Fast Food Establishments								
5. Troublesome Foods								
6. Eat Until Full or Overfull								
7. Candy								
8. Coffee								
9. Non-diet Cola Drinks								
10. Alcohol								
11. Doughnuts								
12. Salad Dressings								
13. Lack of Home Support								
14. Restaurants								
15. Big Meals								
16. Unaware of Food Consumption								
17. Too Much Red Meat								
18. Craving Certain Food								
19. Social Events								
20. Desserts								
21. No Exercise								
22. Lack of Friendly Support								
23. Lack of Motivation								

Now rank the three problems that you feel are contributing most to your tendency to overeat.

1. ______________________________

2. ______________________________

3. ______________________________

YOUR 8-STEP PERSONAL ACTION PLAN

Each week you will design your own individual Personal Action Plan. This plan, designed by you, consists of weight loss goals and strategies for the next week.

1. Weigh yourself and plot your weight on the Weight Loss Profile Sheet (p. 158).
2. Review your Eating and Exercise Diary and Problem Inventory for the week. Identify any problem eating behaviors that need to be corrected.
3. Select one problem eating behavior and describe it in this week's Personal Action Plan (as shown on the following page).
4. Write down several strategies that you could use to alter this selected problem eating behavior. From these strategies, select a best strategy as a solution and include this strategy in next week's Eating and Exercise Diary. Write the strategy in the space provided at the top of next week's Eating and Exercise Diary.
5. Consult with your partner in planning your complete program for the next week.
6. Plan your daily meal and exercise schedules for next week.
7. Indicate your commitment to the weekly Plan of Action by writing a personal statement of commitment.
8. Develop appropriate rewards for successful completion of the selected strategy.

PERSONAL ACTION PLAN

I. **Problem:** ______________________________

____

____

____

II. **Strategies for the Problem**

____

____

____

____

III. **Best Strategy for the Problem**

____

____

____

____

IV. **Weekly Reward**

____

____

____

____

V. **Statement of Commitment**

____

____

____

____

Self-Understanding Exercises

Communication Skills

Assertive Requests

1. Being assertive is following through on my real feelings, wishes, and goals while remaining sensitive to the feelings of others.
2. I have the right to tell other people my feelings and needs as long as I don't violate the rights of others.
3. I can't expect other people to read my mind and know my needs and wants.
4. When I am assertive, there is no guarantee that I will get what I want, but it does create an opportunity for fair negotiations.
5. With practice I can develop the skills necessary for politely requesting what I want and need.
6. The more I practice being directive in my requesting, the more likely I will develop a personality that is assertive.

This week, attempt to make at least five assertive requests to people with whom you have contact.

Refusing Requests

1. Being assertive is following through on my real feelings, wishes, and goals while remaining sensitive to the feelings of others.
2. When I say no, it does not mean that I am rejecting another person; I am simply refusing a request.
3. I always reserve the right to say "no."
4. I must be direct, concise and to the point whenever I say "no."
5. If I really mean "no," I will not allow myself to be manipulated by pleading, begging, cajoling, compliments or other forms of manipulation.
6. I will not apologize for saying "no."
7. Learning to say "no" assertively and not feeling guilty about it can become an important skill in my daily life.

Practice refusing a request five times this week.

Week 4

Daily Food and Exercise Diary

Day of Week ______________________________

Strategy for the Week ______________________

Daily Caloric Quota Reminder	**Daily Fat Gram Budget**

Time	Food	Quantity	Meal or Snack	Where Consumed	Feelings Before Eating	Calories	Fat in Grams

1. Did you eat something from each of the 4 basic food groups? **Yes / No**
   Milk ___ Meat ___ Fruit & Vegetable ___ Grains ___
2. Did you consume most of your food before 2:00 p.m.? **Yes / No**
3. Did you eat all of your food at the same designated place? **Yes / No**
4. Did you stay ± 200 calories of your caloric quota? **Yes / No**
5. Did you stay ± 5 grams of your fat gram budget? **Yes / No**
6. Did you have a planned exercise time for the day? **Yes / No**

If yes: Type ______________________________

Duration ______________________________

Approximate Heart Rate ______________________

Week 4

Daily Food and Exercise Diary

Day of Week ______________________________

Strategy for the Week ______________________

Daily Caloric Quota Reminder

Daily Fat Gram Budget

Time	Food	Quantity	Meal or Snack	Where Consumed	Feelings Before Eating	Calories	Fat in Grams

1. Did you eat something from each of the 4 basic food groups? **Yes / No**
   Milk ___ Meat ___ Fruit & Vegetable ___ Grains ___
2. Did you consume most of your food before 2:00 p.m.? **Yes / No**
3. Did you eat all of your food at the same designated place? **Yes / No**
4. Did you stay ± 200 calories of your caloric quota? **Yes / No**
5. Did you stay ± 5 grams of your fat gram budget? **Yes / No**
6. Did you have a planned exercise time for the day? **Yes / No**

   If yes: Type ______________________________

   Duration ______________________________

   Approximate Heart Rate ______________________

WEEK 4

DAILY FOOD AND EXERCISE DIARY

Day of Week ______________________

Strategy for the Week ______________________

Daily Caloric Quota Reminder	Daily Fat Gram Budget

Time	Food	Quantity	Meal or Snack	Where Consumed	Feelings Before Eating	Calories	Fat in Grams

1. Did you eat something from each of the 4 basic food groups? **Yes / No**
   Milk ___ Meat ___ Fruit & Vegetable ___ Grains ___
2. Did you consume most of your food before 2:00 p.m.? **Yes / No**
3. Did you eat all of your food at the same designated place? **Yes / No**
4. Did you stay $\pm$ 200 calories of your caloric quota? **Yes / No**
5. Did you stay $\pm$ 5 grams of your fat gram budget? **Yes / No**
6. Did you have a planned exercise time for the day? **Yes / No**

If yes: Type ______________________

Duration ______________________

Approximate Heart Rate ______________________

WEEK 4

DAILY FOOD AND EXERCISE DIARY

Day of Week ______________________________

Strategy for the Week ______________________

Daily Caloric Quota Reminder [ ]

Daily Fat Gram Budget [ ]

Time	Food	Quantity	Meal or Snack	Where Consumed	Feelings Before Eating	Calories	Fat in Grams

1. Did you eat something from each of the 4 basic food groups? **Yes / No**
   Milk ___ Meat ___ Fruit & Vegetable ___ Grains ___
2. Did you consume most of your food before 2:00 p.m.? **Yes / No**
3. Did you eat all of your food at the same designated place? **Yes / No**
4. Did you stay ± 200 calories of your caloric quota? **Yes / No**
5. Did you stay ± 5 grams of your fat gram budget? **Yes / No**
6. Did you have a planned exercise time for the day? **Yes / No**

   If yes: Type ______________________________

   Duration ______________________________

   Approximate Heart Rate ______________________

WEEK 4

DAILY FOOD AND EXERCISE DIARY

Day of Week ____________________

Strategy for the Week ____________________

Daily Caloric Quota Reminder	Daily Fat Gram Budget

Time	Food	Quantity	Meal or Snack	Where Consumed	Feelings Before Eating	Calories	Fat in Grams

1. Did you eat something from each of the 4 basic food groups? **Yes / No**
   Milk ___ Meat ___ Fruit & Vegetable ___ Grains ___
2. Did you consume most of your food before 2:00 p.m.? **Yes / No**
3. Did you eat all of your food at the same designated place? **Yes / No**
4. Did you stay ± 200 calories of your caloric quota? **Yes / No**
5. Did you stay ± 5 grams of your fat gram budget? **Yes / No**
6. Did you have a planned exercise time for the day? **Yes / No**

   If yes: Type ____________________

   Duration ____________________

   Approximate Heart Rate ____________________

WEEK 4

DAILY FOOD AND EXERCISE DIARY

Day of Week ______________________

Strategy for the Week ______________________

Daily Caloric Quota Reminder	Daily Fat Gram Budget

Time	Food	Quantity	Meal or Snack	Where Consumed	Feelings Before Eating	Calories	Fat in Grams

1. Did you eat something from each of the 4 basic food groups? **Yes / No**
   Milk ___ Meat ___ Fruit & Vegetable ___ Grains ___
2. Did you consume most of your food before 2:00 p.m.? **Yes / No**
3. Did you eat all of your food at the same designated place? **Yes / No**
4. Did you stay $\pm$ 200 calories of your caloric quota? **Yes / No**
5. Did you stay $\pm$ 5 grams of your fat gram budget? **Yes / No**
6. Did you have a planned exercise time for the day? **Yes / No**

   If yes: Type ______________________

   Duration ______________________

   Approximate Heart Rate ______________________

WEEK 4

DAILY FOOD AND EXERCISE DIARY

Day of Week ______________________________

Strategy for the Week ______________________

Daily Caloric Quota Reminder [ ]

Daily Fat Gram Budget [ ]

Time	Food	Quantity	Meal or Snack	Where Consumed	Feelings Before Eating	Calories	Fat in Grams

1. Did you eat something from each of the 4 basic food groups? **Yes / No**
   Milk ___ Meat ___ Fruit & Vegetable ___ Grains ___
2. Did you consume most of your food before 2:00 p.m.? **Yes / No**
3. Did you eat all of your food at the same designated place? **Yes / No**
4. Did you stay ± 200 calories of your caloric quota? **Yes / No**
5. Did you stay ± 5 grams of your fat gram budget? **Yes / No**
6. Did you have a planned exercise time for the day? **Yes / No**

If yes: Type ______________________________

Duration ______________________________

Approximate Heart Rate ______________________

PROBLEM INVENTORY FOR THE WEEK

Each day check those items that you perceive as problems that make you want to overeat. At the end of the week, total the number of days during the week each item was a problem.	M	T	W	T	F	S	S	TOTAL
1. Snacks								
2. High Fat								
3. Sugar								
4. Fast Food Establishments								
5. Troublesome Foods								
6. Eat Until Full or Overfull								
7. Candy								
8. Coffee								
9. Non-diet Cola Drinks								
10. Alcohol								
11. Doughnuts								
12. Salad Dressings								
13. Lack of Home Support								
14. Restaurants								
15. Big Meals								
16. Unaware of Food Consumption								
17. Too Much Red Meat								
18. Craving Certain Food								
19. Social Events								
20. Desserts								
21. No Exercise								
22. Lack of Friendly Support								
23. Lack of Motivation								

Now rank the three problems that you feel are contributing most to your tendency to overeat.

1. ______________________________
2. ______________________________
3. ______________________________

YOUR 8-STEP PERSONAL ACTION PLAN

Each week you will design your own individual Personal Action Plan. This plan, designed by you, consists of weight loss goals and strategies for the next week.

1. Weigh yourself and plot your weight on the Weight Loss Profile Sheet (p. 158).
2. Review your Eating and Exercise Diary and Problem Inventory for the week. Identify any problem eating behaviors that need to be corrected.
3. Select one problem eating behavior and describe it in this week's Personal Action Plan (as shown on the following page).
4. Write down several strategies that you could use to alter this selected problem eating behavior. From these strategies, select a best strategy as a solution and include this strategy in next week's Eating and Exercise Diary. Write the strategy in the space provided at the top of next week's Eating and Exercise Diary.
5. Consult with your partner in planning your complete program for the next week.
6. Plan your daily meal and exercise schedules for next week.
7. Indicate your commitment to the weekly Plan of Action by writing a personal statement of commitment.
8. Develop appropriate rewards for successful completion of the selected strategy.

Personal Action Plan

I. **Problem:** ______________________________

____

____

____

II. **Strategies for the Problem**

____

____

____

____

III. **Best Strategy for the Problem**

____

____

____

____

IV. **Weekly Reward**

____

____

____

____

V. **Statement of Commitment**

____

____

____

____

WEEK 5

UNDERSTANDING YOUR FEELINGS

It is important to know yourself and your feelings. Feelings may be the major cause of your overeating problem. With an understanding of the feelings that sometimes cause you to eat, you can take control of the events that produce these feelings.

Using the key lists below, write down your feelings and the intensity of these feelings before eating a meal or snack. Be certain to include feelings not listed on this key.

Feeling Key

A = angry	F = frustrated
B = bored	H = happy
C = craving	R = rushed
D = depressed	S = stable or neutral
E = excited	T = tired

* Other feelings

Intensity

1 = mild
2 = moderate
3 = extreme

Time	M	T	W	TH	F	S	SU
6:00 am							
10:00 am							
2:00 pm							
6:00 pm							
10:00 pm							

WEEK 5

DAILY FOOD AND EXERCISE DIARY

Day of Week ______________________

Strategy for the Week ______________________

Daily Caloric Quota Reminder	**Daily Fat Gram Budget**

Time	Food	Quantity	Meal or Snack	Where Consumed	Feelings Before Eating	Calories	Fat in Grams

1. Did you eat something from each of the 4 basic food groups? **Yes / No**
   Milk ___ Meat ___ Fruit & Vegetable ___ Grains ___
2. Did you consume most of your food before 2:00 p.m.? **Yes / No**
3. Did you eat all of your food at the same designated place? **Yes / No**
4. Did you stay $\pm$200 calories of your caloric quota? **Yes / No**
5. Did you stay $\pm$ 5 grams of your fat gram budget? **Yes / No**
6. Did you have a planned exercise time for the day? **Yes / No**

If yes: Type ______________________

Duration ______________________

Approximate Heart Rate ______________________

WEEK 5

DAILY FOOD AND EXERCISE DIARY

Day of Week ______________________________

Strategy for the Week ______________________

Daily Caloric Quota Reminder	Daily Fat Gram Budget

Time	Food	Quantity	Meal or Snack	Where Consumed	Feelings Before Eating	Calories	Fat in Grams

1. Did you eat something from each of the 4 basic food groups? **Yes / No**
   Milk ___ Meat ___ Fruit & Vegetable ___ Grains ___
2. Did you consume most of your food before 2:00 p.m.? **Yes / No**
3. Did you eat all of your food at the same designated place? **Yes / No**
4. Did you stay ± 200 calories of your caloric quota? **Yes / No**
5. Did you stay ± 5 grams of your fat gram budget? **Yes / No**
6. Did you have a planned exercise time for the day? **Yes / No**

   If yes: Type ______________________________________

   Duration ___________________________________

   Approximate Heart Rate ______________________

WEEK 5

DAILY FOOD AND EXERCISE DIARY

Day of Week ______________________

Strategy for the Week ______________________

Daily Caloric Quota Reminder	Daily Fat Gram Budget

Time	Food	Quantity	Meal or Snack	Where Consumed	Feelings Before Eating	Calories	Fat In Grams

1. Did you eat something from each of the 4 basic food groups? **Yes / No**
   Milk ___ Meat ___ Fruit & Vegetable ___ Grains ___
2. Did you consume most of your food before 2:00 p.m.? **Yes / No**
3. Did you eat all of your food at the same designated place? **Yes / No**
4. Did you stay ± 200 calories of your caloric quota? **Yes / No**
5. Did you stay ± 5 grams of your fat gram budget? **Yes / No**
6. Did you have a planned exercise time for the day? **Yes / No**

   If yes: Type ______________________

   Duration ______________________

   Approximate Heart Rate ______________________

DAILY FOOD AND EXERCISE DIARY

Day of Week ______________________

Strategy for the Week ______________________

Daily Caloric Quota Reminder	**Daily Fat Gram Budget**

Time	Food	Quantity	Meal or Snack	Where Consumed	Feelings Before Eating	Calories	Fat in Grams

1. Did you eat something from each of the 4 basic food groups? **Yes / No**
   Milk ___ Meat ___ Fruit & Vegetable ___ Grains ___
2. Did you consume most of your food before 2:00 p.m.? **Yes / No**
3. Did you eat all of your food at the same designated place? **Yes / No**
4. Did you stay ± 200 calories of your caloric quota? **Yes / No**
5. Did you stay ± 5 grams of your fat gram budget? **Yes / No**
6. Did you have a planned exercise time for the day? **Yes / No**

If yes: Type ______________________

Duration ______________________

Approximate Heart Rate ______________________

WEEK 5

DAILY FOOD AND EXERCISE DIARY

Day of Week ______________________

Strategy for the Week ______________________

Daily Caloric Quota Reminder [ ]

Daily Fat Gram Budget [ ]

Time	Food	Quantity	Meal or Snack	Where Consumed	Feelings Before Eating	Calories	Fat in Grams

1. Did you eat something from each of the 4 basic food groups? **Yes / No**
   Milk ___ Meat ___ Fruit & Vegetable ___ Grains ___
2. Did you consume most of your food before 2:00 p.m.? **Yes / No**
3. Did you eat all of your food at the same designated place? **Yes / No**
4. Did you stay ± 200 calories of your caloric quota? **Yes / No**
5. Did you stay ± 5 grams of your fat gram budget? **Yes / No**
6. Did you have a planned exercise time for the day? **Yes / No**

   If yes: Type ______________________

   Duration ______________________

   Approximate Heart Rate ______________________

Week 5

Daily Food and Exercise Diary

Day of Week ______________________________

Strategy for the Week ______________________

Daily Caloric Quota Reminder	**Daily Fat Gram Budget**

Time	Food	Quantity	Meal or Snack	Where Consumed	Feelings Before Eating	Calories	Fat in Grams

1. Did you eat something from each of the 4 basic food groups? **Yes / No**
   Milk ___ Meat ___ Fruit & Vegetable ___ Grains ___
2. Did you consume most of your food before 2:00 p.m.? **Yes / No**
3. Did you eat all of your food at the same designated place? **Yes / No**
4. Did you stay ± 200 calories of your caloric quota? **Yes / No**
5. Did you stay ± 5 grams of your fat gram budget? **Yes / No**
6. Did you have a planned exercise time for the day? **Yes / No**

   If yes: Type ______________________________

   Duration ______________________________

   Approximate Heart Rate ______________________

DAILY FOOD AND EXERCISE DIARY

Day of Week ____________________

Strategy for the Week ____________________

Daily Caloric Quota Reminder	**Daily Fat Gram Budget**

Time	Food	Quantity	Meal or Snack	Where Consumed	Feelings Before Eating	Calories	Fat in Grams

1. Did you eat something from each of the 4 basic food groups? **Yes / No**
   Milk ___ Meat ___ Fruit & Vegetable ___ Grains ___
2. Did you consume most of your food before 2:00 p.m.? **Yes / No**
3. Did you eat all of your food at the same designated place? **Yes / No**
4. Did you stay ± 200 calories of your caloric quota? **Yes / No**
5. Did you stay ± 5 grams of your fat gram budget? **Yes / No**
6. Did you have a planned exercise time for the day? **Yes / No**

   If yes: Type ____________________

   Duration ____________________

   Approximate Heart Rate ____________________

WEEK 5

PROBLEM INVENTORY FOR THE WEEK

Each day check those items that you perceive as problems that make you want to overeat. At the end of the week, total the number of days during the week each item was a problem.	M	T	W	T	F	S	S	TOTAL
1. Snacks								
2. High Fat								
3. Sugar								
4. Fast Food Establishments								
5. Troublesome Foods								
6. Eat Until Full or Overfull								
7. Candy								
8. Coffee								
9. Non-diet Cola Drinks								
10. Alcohol								
11. Doughnuts								
12. Salad Dressings								
13. Lack of Home Support								
14. Restaurants								
15. Big Meals								
16. Unaware of Food Consumption								
17. Too Much Red Meat								
18. Craving Certain Food								
19. Social Events								
20. Desserts								
21. No Exercise								
22. Lack of Friendly Support								
23. Lack of Motivation								

Now rank the three problems that you feel are contributing most to your tendency to overeat.

1. ______________________________

2. ______________________________

3. ______________________________

YOUR 8-STEP PERSONAL ACTION PLAN

Each week you will design your own individual Personal Action Plan. This plan, designed by you, consists of weight loss goals and strategies for the next week.

1. Weigh yourself and plot your weight on the Weight Loss Profile Sheet (p. 158).
2. Review your Eating and Exercise Diary and Problem Inventory for the week. Identify any problem eating behaviors that need to be corrected.
3. Select one problem eating behavior and describe it in this week's Personal Action Plan (as shown on the following page).
4. Write down several strategies that you could use to alter this selected problem eating behavior. From these strategies, select a best strategy as a solution and include this strategy in next week's Eating and Exercise Diary. Write the strategy in the space provided at the top of next week's Eating and Exercise Diary.
5. Consult with your partner in planning your complete program for the next week.
6. Plan your daily meal and exercise schedules for next week.
7. Indicate your commitment to the weekly Plan of Action by writing a personal statement of commitment.
8. Develop appropriate rewards for successful completion of the selected strategy.

Personal Action Plan

I. **Problem:** ______________________________

____

____

____

II. **Strategies for the Problem**

____

____

____

____

III. **Best Strategy for the Problem**

____

____

____

____

IV. **Weekly Reward**

____

____

____

____

V. **Statement of Commitment**

____

____

____

____

Week 6

Understanding When You Eat

Becoming aware of **when you eat** is an important step in modifying your food intake. Do you eat most of your food in the morning? Do you come home in the afternoon and eat everything in sight? Are you a late night snacker? By doing the following exercise you can become more aware of your daily eating patterns during the week. In each time segment indicate if you ate a meal (M) or snack (S). Changing your food consumption to a time that corresponds with more physical activity is an important step toward permanent weight control.

Indicate Meal (M) or Snack (S) (For each time span)

Time	M	T	W	TH	F	S	SU	Total Calories
6:00 a.m								
10:00 a.m.								
2:00 p.m.								
6:00 p.m.								
10:00 a.m.								

DAILY FOOD AND EXERCISE DIARY

Day of Week ______________________

Strategy for the Week ________________

Daily Caloric Quota Reminder [ ]

Daily Fat Gram Budget [ ]

Time	Food	Quantity	Meal or Snack	Where Consumed	Feelings Before Eating	Calories	Fat in Grams

1. Did you eat something from each of the 4 basic food groups? **Yes / No**
   Milk ___ Meat ___ Fruit & Vegetable ___ Grains ___
2. Did you consume most of your food before 2:00 p.m.? **Yes / No**
3. Did you eat all of your food at the same designated place? **Yes / No**
4. Did you stay $\pm$ 200 calories of your caloric quota? **Yes / No**
5. Did you stay $\pm$ 5 grams of your fat gram budget? **Yes / No**
6. Did you have a planned exercise time for the day? **Yes / No**

If yes: Type ______________________

Duration ______________________

Approximate Heart Rate ______________________

Week 6

Daily Food and Exercise Diary

Day of Week ____________________

Strategy for the Week ____________________

Daily Caloric Quota Reminder	**Daily Fat Gram Budget**

Time	Food	Quantity	Meal or Snack	Where Consumed	Feelings Before Eating	Calories	Fat in Grams

1. Did you eat something from each of the 4 basic food groups? **Yes / No**
   Milk ___ Meat ___ Fruit & Vegetable ___ Grains ___
2. Did you consume most of your food before 2:00 p.m.? **Yes / No**
3. Did you eat all of your food at the same designated place? **Yes / No**
4. Did you stay ± 200 calories of your caloric quota? **Yes / No**
5. Did you stay ± 5 grams of your fat gram budget? **Yes / No**
6. Did you have a planned exercise time for the day? **Yes / No**

If yes: Type ____________________

Duration ____________________

Approximate Heart Rate ____________________

Week 6

Daily Food and Exercise Diary

Day of Week ______________________________

Strategy for the Week ______________________

Daily Caloric Quota Reminder	**Daily Fat Gram Budget**

Time	Food	Quantity	Meal or Snack	Where Consumed	Feelings Before Eating	Calories	Fat in Grams

1. Did you eat something from each of the 4 basic food groups? **Yes / No**
   Milk___ Meat___ Fruit & Vegetable___ Grains___
2. Did you consume most of your food before 2:00 p.m.? **Yes / No**
3. Did you eat all of your food at the same designated place? **Yes / No**
4. Did you stay ± 200 calories of your caloric quota? **Yes / No**
5. Did you stay ± 5 grams of your fat gram budget? **Yes / No**
6. Did you have a planned exercise time for the day? **Yes / No**

   If yes: Type ______________________________

   Duration ______________________________

   Approximate Heart Rate ______________________

WEEK 6

DAILY FOOD AND EXERCISE DIARY

Day of Week ______________________________

Strategy for the Week ______________________

Daily Caloric Quota Reminder	Daily Fat Gram Budget

Time	Food	Quantity	Meal or Snack	Where Consumed	Feelings Before Eating	Calories	Fat in Grams

1. Did you eat something from each of the 4 basic food groups? **Yes / No**
   Milk ___ Meat ___ Fruit & Vegetable ___ Grains ___
2. Did you consume most of your food before 2:00 p.m.? **Yes / No**
3. Did you eat all of your food at the same designated place? **Yes / No**
4. Did you stay ± 200 calories of your caloric quota? **Yes / No**
5. Did you stay ± 5 grams of your fat gram budget? **Yes / No**
6. Did you have a planned exercise time for the day? **Yes / No**

   If yes: Type ______________________________

   Duration ______________________________

   Approximate Heart Rate ______________________

WEEK 6

DAILY FOOD AND EXERCISE DIARY

Day of Week ______________________

Strategy for the Week ______________________

Daily Caloric Quota Reminder	Daily Fat Gram Budget

Time	Food	Quantity	Meal or Snack	Where Consumed	Feelings Before Eating	Calories	Fat in Grams

1. Did you eat something from each of the 4 basic food groups? **Yes / No**
   Milk ___ Meat ___ Fruit & Vegetable ___ Grains ___
2. Did you consume most of your food before 2:00 p.m.? **Yes / No**
3. Did you eat all of your food at the same designated place? **Yes / No**
4. Did you stay ± 200 calories of your caloric quota? **Yes / No**
5. Did you stay ± 5 grams of your fat gram budget? **Yes / No**
6. Did you have a planned exercise time for the day? **Yes / No**

   If yes: Type ______________________

   Duration ______________________

   Approximate Heart Rate ______________________

WEEK 6

DAILY FOOD AND EXERCISE DIARY

Day of Week ______________________________

Strategy for the Week ______________________

Daily Caloric Quota Reminder	Daily Fat Gram Budget

Time	Food	Quantity	Meal or Snack	Where Consumed	Feelings Before Eating	Calories	Fat in Grams

1. Did you eat something from each of the 4 basic food groups? **Yes / No**
   Milk___ Meat___ Fruit & Vegetable___ Grains___
2. Did you consume most of your food before 2:00 p.m.? **Yes / No**
3. Did you eat all of your food at the same designated place? **Yes / No**
4. Did you stay ± 200 calories of your caloric quota? **Yes / No**
5. Did you stay ± 5 grams of your fat gram budget? **Yes / No**
6. Did you have a planned exercise time for the day? **Yes / No**

   If yes: Type ____________________________________

   Duration ____________________________________

   Approximate Heart Rate ________________________

WEEK 6

DAILY FOOD AND EXERCISE DIARY

Day of Week ______________________________

Strategy for the Week ______________________

Daily Caloric Quota Reminder [ ]

Daily Fat Gram Budget [ ]

Time	Food	Quantity	Meal or Snack	Where Consumed	Feelings Before Eating	Calories	Fat in Grams

1. Did you eat something from each of the 4 basic food groups? **Yes / No**
   Milk ___ Meat ___ Fruit & Vegetable ___ Grains ___
2. Did you consume most of your food before 2:00 p.m.? **Yes / No**
3. Did you eat all of your food at the same designated place? **Yes / No**
4. Did you stay ± 200 calories of your caloric quota? **Yes / No**
5. Did you stay ± 5 grams of your fat gram budget? **Yes / No**
6. Did you have a planned exercise time for the day? **Yes / No**

   If yes: Type ______________________________

   Duration ______________________________

   Approximate Heart Rate ______________________

PROBLEM INVENTORY FOR THE WEEK

Each day check those items that you perceive as problems that make you want to overeat. At the end of the week, total the number of days during the week each item was a problem.

	M	T	W	T	F	S	S	TOTAL
1. Snacks								
2. High Fat								
3. Sugar								
4. Fast Food Establishments								
5. Troublesome Foods								
6. Eat Until Full or Overfull								
7. Candy								
8. Coffee								
9. Non-diet Cola Drinks								
10. Alcohol								
11. Doughnuts								
12. Salad Dressings								
13. Lack of Home Support								
14. Restaurants								
15. Big Meals								
16. Unaware of Food Consumption								
17. Too Much Red Meat								
18. Craving Certain Food								
19. Social Events								
20. Desserts								
21. No Exercise								
22. Lack of Friendly Support								
23. Lack of Motivation								

Now rank the three problems that you feel are contributing most to your tendency to overeat.

1. ______________________
2. ______________________
3. ______________________

YOUR 8-STEP PERSONAL ACTION PLAN

Each week you will design your own individual Personal Action Plan. This plan, designed by you, consists of weight loss goals and strategies for the next week.

1. Weigh yourself and plot your weight on the Weight Loss Profile Sheet (p. 158).
2. Review your Eating and Exercise Diary and Problem Inventory for the week. Identify any problem eating behaviors that need to be corrected.
3. Select one problem eating behavior and describe it in this week's Personal Action Plan (as shown on the following page).
4. Write down several strategies that you could use to alter this selected problem eating behavior. From these strategies, select a best strategy as a solution and include this strategy in next week's Eating and Exercise Diary. Write the strategy in the space provided at the top of next week's Eating and Exercise Diary.
5. Consult with your partner in planning your complete program for the next week.
6. Plan your daily meal and exercise schedules for next week.
7. Indicate your commitment to the weekly Plan of Action by writing a personal statement of commitment.
8. Develop appropriate rewards for successful completion of the selected strategy.

Personal Action Plan

I. **Problem:** ______________________________

____

____

____

II. **Strategies for the Problem**

____

____

____

____

III. **Best Strategy for the Problem**

____

____

____

____

IV. **Weekly Reward**

____

____

____

____

V. **Statement of Commitment**

____

____

____

____

Self-Understanding Exercises

Assertiveness and Weight Control

What is your response to the following questions? Plan strategies based on the communication skills mentioned in the previous exercise for each of the following situations.

1. "Have a slice of this pie—I made it especially for you."
2. "You aren't eating. Don't you like my cooking?"
3. "Let's jump in the car and go get a hamburger and some fries."
4. "I don't like it when you diet."
5. "Make mine a double. I don't like to drink alone."
6. "Here, have some. It's O.K. It's the holidays."
7. "Try some of this. You can get back on your diet tomorrow."
8. "Eat the rest of this. I hate to see it go to waste."
9. "You aren't eating much. Is something bothering you?"
10. "If you don't eat, you'll get sick."
11. "I made this just for you; it's your favorite."
12. "Are you sure you don't want seconds?"

DESIGNATED EATING PLACE

Knowing where you eat most of your food is important. By filling in the following chart you will be able to see how your eating is related to being in certain places and how your environment may stimulate you to overeat. Your goal is to gradually modify this eating pattern and eventually eat most of your food in one specific place.

Each time you eat, indicate if it is a Meal (M) or Snack(S) and write it in by the eating locations listed below.

Places	M	T	W	TH	F	S	SU
Cafeteria							
Den/Living Room							
Car							
Kitchen table							
Restaurant							
Fast food place							
Kitchen							
Bedroom							
Break room							
____________							
____________							
____________							

WEEK 7

DAILY FOOD AND EXERCISE DIARY

Day of Week ______________________________

Strategy for the Week ______________________

Daily Caloric Quota Reminder [ ]

Daily Fat Gram Budget [ ]

Time	Food	Quantity	Meal or Snack	Where Consumed	Feelings Before Eating	Calories	Fat in Grams

1. Did you eat something from each of the 4 basic food groups? **Yes / No**
   Milk ___ Meat ___ Fruit & Vegetable ___ Grains ___
2. Did you consume most of your food before 2:00 p.m.? **Yes / No**
3. Did you eat all of your food at the same designated place? **Yes / No**
4. Did you stay ± 200 calories of your caloric quota? **Yes / No**
5. Did you stay ± 5 grams of your fat gram budget? **Yes / No**
6. Did you have a planned exercise time for the day? **Yes / No**

If yes: Type ______________________________

Duration ______________________________

Approximate Heart Rate ______________________

WEEK 7

DAILY FOOD AND EXERCISE DIARY

Day of Week ______________________

Strategy for the Week ______________________

Daily Caloric Quota Reminder	Daily Fat Gram Budget

Time	Food	Quantity	Meal or Snack	Where Consumed	Feelings Before Eating	Calories	Fat in Grams

1. Did you eat something from each of the 4 basic food groups? Yes / No
   Milk ___ Meat ___ Fruit & Vegetable ___ Grains ___
2. Did you consume most of your food before 2:00 p.m.? Yes / No
3. Did you eat all of your food at the same designated place? Yes / No
4. Did you stay ± 200 calories of your caloric quota? Yes / No
5. Did you stay ± 5 grams of your fat gram budget? Yes / No
6. Did you have a planned exercise time for the day? Yes / No

   If yes: Type ______________________

   Duration ______________________

   Approximate Heart Rate ______________________

Week 7

Daily Food and Exercise Diary

Day of Week ______________________________

Strategy for the Week ______________________

Daily Caloric Quota Reminder [ ]

Daily Fat Gram Budget [ ]

Time	Food	Quantity	Meal or Snack	Where Consumed	Feelings Before Eating	Calories	Fat in Grams

1. Did you eat something from each of the 4 basic food groups? **Yes / No**
   Milk ___ Meat ___ Fruit & Vegetable ___ Grains ___
2. Did you consume most of your food before 2:00 p.m.? **Yes / No**
3. Did you eat all of your food at the same designated place? **Yes / No**
4. Did you stay $\pm$200 calories of your caloric quota? **Yes / No**
5. Did you stay $\pm$5 grams of your fat gram budget? **Yes / No**
6. Did you have a planned exercise time for the day? **Yes / No**

If yes: Type ______________________________

Duration ______________________________

Approximate Heart Rate ______________________

WEEK 7

DAILY FOOD AND EXERCISE DIARY

Day of Week ______________________________

Strategy for the Week ______________________

Daily Caloric Quota Reminder [ ]

Daily Fat Gram Budget [ ]

Time	Food	Quantity	Meal or Snack	Where Consumed	Feelings Before Eating	Calories	Fat in Grams

1. Did you eat something from each of the 4 basic food groups? **Yes / No**
   Milk ___ Meat ___ Fruit & Vegetable ___ Grains ___
2. Did you consume most of your food before 2:00 p.m.? **Yes / No**
3. Did you eat all of your food at the same designated place? **Yes / No**
4. Did you stay ±200 calories of your caloric quota? **Yes / No**
5. Did you stay ± 5 grams of your fat gram budget? **Yes / No**
6. Did you have a planned exercise time for the day? **Yes / No**

If yes: Type ______________________________

Duration ______________________________

Approximate Heart Rate ______________________

WEEK 7

DAILY FOOD AND EXERCISE DIARY

Day of Week ______________________

Strategy for the Week ______________________

Daily Caloric Quota Reminder [ ]

Daily Fat Gram Budget [ ]

Time	Food	Quantity	Meal or Snack	Where Consumed	Feelings Before Eating	Calories	Fat in Grams

1. Did you eat something from each of the 4 basic food groups? **Yes / No**
   Milk ___ Meat ___ Fruit & Vegetable ___ Grains ___
2. Did you consume most of your food before 2:00 p.m.? **Yes / No**
3. Did you eat all of your food at the same designated place? **Yes / No**
4. Did you stay ± 200 calories of your caloric quota? **Yes / No**
5. Did you stay ± 5 grams of your fat gram budget? **Yes / No**
6. Did you have a planned exercise time for the day? **Yes / No**

If yes: Type ______________________

Duration ______________________

Approximate Heart Rate ______________________

WEEK 7

DAILY FOOD AND EXERCISE DIARY

Day of Week ___________________________

Strategy for the Week ____________________

Daily Caloric Quota Reminder

Daily Fat Gram Budget

Time	Food	Quantity	Meal or Snack	Where Consumed	Feelings Before Eating	Calories	Fat in Grams

1. Did you eat something from each of the 4 basic food groups? **Yes / No**
   Milk ___ Meat ___ Fruit & Vegetable ___ Grains ___
2. Did you consume most of your food before 2:00 p.m.? **Yes / No**
3. Did you eat all of your food at the same designated place? **Yes / No**
4. Did you stay ± 200 calories of your caloric quota? **Yes / No**
5. Did you stay ± 5 grams of your fat gram budget? **Yes / No**
6. Did you have a planned exercise time for the day? **Yes / No**

   If yes: Type ___________________________

   Duration ___________________________

   Approximate Heart Rate ____________________

WEEK 7

DAILY FOOD AND EXERCISE DIARY

Day of Week ____________________________

Strategy for the Week ______________________

Daily Caloric Quota Reminder	Daily Fat Gram Budget

Time	Food	Quantity	Meal or Snack	Where Consumed	Feelings Before Eating	Calories	Fat in Grams

1. Did you eat something from each of the 4 basic food groups? **Yes / No**
   Milk___ Meat___ Fruit & Vegetable___ Grains___
2. Did you consume most of your food before 2:00 p.m.? **Yes / No**
3. Did you eat all of your food at the same designated place? **Yes / No**
4. Did you stay ± 200 calories of your caloric quota? **Yes / No**
5. Did you stay ± 5 grams of your fat gram budget? **Yes / No**
6. Did you have a planned exercise time for the day? **Yes / No**

If yes: Type ______________________________

Duration ______________________________

Approximate Heart Rate ______________________

PROBLEM INVENTORY FOR THE WEEK

Each day check those items that you perceive as problems that make you want to overeat. At the end of the week, total the number of days during the week each item was a problem.

	M	T	W	T	F	S	S	TOTAL
1. Snacks								
2. High Fat								
3. Sugar								
4. Fast Food Establishments								
5. Troublesome Foods								
6. Eat Until Full or Overfull								
7. Candy								
8. Coffee								
9. Non-diet Cola Drinks								
10. Alcohol								
11. Doughnuts								
12. Salad Dressings								
13. Lack of Home Support								
14. Restaurants								
15. Big Meals								
16. Unaware of Food Consumption								
17. Too Much Red Meat								
18. Craving Certain Food								
19. Social Events								
20. Desserts								
21. No Exercise								
22. Lack of Friendly Support								
23. Lack of Motivation								

Now rank the three problems that you feel are contributing most to your tendency to overeat.

1. ______________________________
2. ______________________________
3. ______________________________

YOUR 8-STEP PERSONAL ACTION PLAN

Each week you will design your own individual Personal Action Plan. This plan, designed by you, consists of weight loss goals and strategies for the next week.

1. Weigh yourself and plot your weight on the Weight Loss Profile Sheet (p. 158).
2. Review your Eating and Exercise Diary and Problem Inventory for the week. Identify any problem eating behaviors that need to be corrected.
3. Select one problem eating behavior and describe it in this week's Personal Action Plan (as shown on the following page).
4. Write down several strategies that you could use to alter this selected problem eating behavior. From these strategies, select a best strategy as a solution and include this strategy in next week's Eating and Exercise Diary. Write the strategy in the space provided at the top of next week's Eating and Exercise Diary.
5. Consult with your partner in planning your complete program for the next week.
6. Plan your daily meal and exercise schedules for next week.
7. Indicate your commitment to the weekly Plan of Action by writing a personal statement of commitment.
8. Develop appropriate rewards for successful completion of the selected strategy.

PERSONAL ACTION PLAN

I. **Problem:** ______________________________

____

____

____

II. **Strategies for the Problem**

____

____

____

____

III. **Best Strategy for the Problem**

____

____

____

____

IV. **Weekly Reward**

____

____

____

____

V. **Statement of Commitment**

____

____

____

____

Self-Understanding Exercises

Suggested Home Relaxation Exercise

(3 to 5 minutes) This short relaxation exercise is excellent for both dieters and nondieters. It provides a brief pause in the day for the person who may eat as the result of anxiety, stress, or other emotional cues. This technique should be practiced throughout the day as needed.

1. Sit comfortably, head held straight, facing forward. While holding your head in this position, look upward towards you eyebrows. Now gaze toward the top of your head. Slowly take a deep breath in and then slowly close your eyelids as you exhale. Return to your normal position. Repeat several times.
2. You should begin to feel relaxed. Release any tension in your head and neck muscles and allow your head to gently roll forward.
3. Next, focus on releasing the tension and relaxing the shoulders and each area of the body (arms, hands, stomach, upper and lower back, buttocks, legs and feet).
4. It is important to control breathing by inhaling and exhaling very slowly and deeply using the abdominal muscles.
5. After relaxing your entire body, try to imagine being in a quiet, pleasant location such as a beach or swimming pool, where you would feel totally at ease. Continue for approximately 2 minutes.
6. Awake refreshed and relaxed.

WEEK 8

DAILY FOOD AND EXERCISE DIARY

Day of Week ______________________________

Strategy for the Week ______________________

Daily Caloric Quota Reminder [ ] **Daily Fat Gram Budget** [ ]

Time	Food	Quantity	Meal or Snack	Where Consumed	Feelings Before Eating	Calories	Fat in Grams

1. Did you eat something from each of the 4 basic food groups? **Yes / No**
   Milk ___ Meat ___ Fruit & Vegetable ___ Grains ___
2. Did you consume most of your food before 2:00 p.m.? **Yes / No**
3. Did you eat all of your food at the same designated place? **Yes / No**
4. Did you stay $\pm$ 200 calories of your caloric quota? **Yes / No**
5. Did you stay $\pm$ 5 grams of your fat gram budget? **Yes / No**
6. Did you have a planned exercise time for the day? **Yes / No**

If yes: Type ______________________________

Duration ______________________________

Approximate Heart Rate ______________________

WEEK 8

DAILY FOOD AND EXERCISE DIARY

Day of Week ______________________________

Strategy for the Week ______________________

Daily Caloric Quota Reminder	Daily Fat Gram Budget

Time	Food	Quantity	Meal or Snack	Where Consumed	Feelings Before Eating	Calories	Fat In Grams

1. Did you eat something from each of the 4 basic food groups? **Yes / No**
   Milk ___ Meat ___ Fruit & Vegetable ___ Grains ___
2. Did you consume most of your food before 2:00 p.m.? **Yes / No**
3. Did you eat all of your food at the same designated place? **Yes / No**
4. Did you stay ±200 calories of your caloric quota? **Yes / No**
5. Did you stay ± 5 grams of your fat gram budget? **Yes / No**
6. Did you have a planned exercise time for the day? **Yes / No**

   If yes: Type ______________________________

   Duration ______________________________

   Approximate Heart Rate ______________________

DAILY FOOD AND EXERCISE DIARY

Day of Week ______________________________

Strategy for the Week ______________________

Daily Caloric Quota Reminder [ ]

Daily Fat Gram Budget [ ]

Time	Food	Quantity	Meal or Snack	Where Consumed	Feelings Before Eating	Calories	Fat in Grams

1. Did you eat something from each of the 4 basic food groups? **Yes / No**
   Milk ___ Meat ___ Fruit & Vegetable ___ Grains ___
2. Did you consume most of your food before 2:00 p.m.? **Yes / No**
3. Did you eat all of your food at the same designated place? **Yes / No**
4. Did you stay ± 200 calories of your caloric quota? **Yes / No**
5. Did you stay ± 5 grams of your fat gram budget? **Yes / No**
6. Did you have a planned exercise time for the day? **Yes / No**

   If yes: Type ______________________________

   Duration ______________________________

   Approximate Heart Rate ______________________

Week 8

Daily Food and Exercise Diary

Day of Week ____________________

Strategy for the Week ____________________

Daily Caloric Quota Reminder	Daily Fat Gram Budget

Time	Food	Quantity	Meal or Snack	Where Consumed	Feelings Before Eating	Calories	Fat in Grams

1. Did you eat something from each of the 4 basic food groups? **Yes / No**
   Milk ___ Meat ___ Fruit & Vegetable ___ Grains ___
2. Did you consume most of your food before 2:00 p.m.? **Yes / No**
3. Did you eat all of your food at the same designated place? **Yes / No**
4. Did you stay ± 200 calories of your caloric quota? **Yes / No**
5. Did you stay ± 5 grams of your fat gram budget? **Yes / No**
6. Did you have a planned exercise time for the day? **Yes / No**

If yes: Type ____________________

Duration ____________________

Approximate Heart Rate ____________________

WEEK 8

DAILY FOOD AND EXERCISE DIARY

Day of Week ______________________

Strategy for the Week ______________________

Daily Caloric Quota Reminder	Daily Fat Gram Budget

Time	Food	Quantity	Meal or Snack	Where Consumed	Feelings Before Eating	Calories	Fat in Grams

1. Did you eat something from each of the 4 basic food groups? **Yes / No**

   Milk ___ Meat ___ Fruit & Vegetable ___ Grains ___
2. Did you consume most of your food before 2:00 p.m.? **Yes / No**
3. Did you eat all of your food at the same designated place? **Yes / No**
4. Did you stay ± 200 calories of your caloric quota? **Yes / No**
5. Did you stay ± 5 grams of your fat gram budget? **Yes / No**
6. Did you have a planned exercise time for the day? **Yes / No**

   If yes: Type ______________________

   Duration ______________________

   Approximate Heart Rate ______________________

WEEK 8

DAILY FOOD AND EXERCISE DIARY

Day of Week ______________________________

Strategy for the Week ______________________

Daily Caloric Quota Reminder	Daily Fat Gram Budget

Time	Food	Quantity	Meal or Snack	Where Consumed	Feelings Before Eating	Calories	Fat in Grams

1. Did you eat something from each of the 4 basic food groups? **Yes / No**
   Milk ___ Meat ___ Fruit & Vegetable ___ Grains ___
2. Did you consume most of your food before 2:00 p.m.? **Yes / No**
3. Did you eat all of your food at the same designated place? **Yes / No**
4. Did you stay ± 200 calories of your caloric quota? **Yes / No**
5. Did you stay ± 5 grams of your fat gram budget? **Yes / No**
6. Did you have a planned exercise time for the day? **Yes / No**

   If yes: Type ______________________________

   Duration ______________________________

   Approximate Heart Rate ______________________

WEEK 8

DAILY FOOD AND EXERCISE DIARY

Day of Week ____________________

Strategy for the Week ____________________

Daily Caloric Quota Reminder	Daily Fat Gram Budget

Time	Food	Quantity	Meal or Snack	Where Consumed	Feelings Before Eating	Calories	Fat in Grams

1. Did you eat something from each of the 4 basic food groups? Yes / No
   Milk ___ Meat ___ Fruit & Vegetable ___ Grains ___
2. Did you consume most of your food before 2:00 p.m.? Yes / No
3. Did you eat all of your food at the same designated place? Yes / No
4. Did you stay ± 200 calories of your caloric quota? Yes / No
5. Did you stay ± 5 grams of your fat gram budget? Yes / No
6. Did you have a planned exercise time for the day? Yes / No

   If yes: Type ____________________

   Duration ____________________

   Approximate Heart Rate ____________________

WEEK 8

PROBLEM INVENTORY FOR THE WEEK

Each day check those items that you perceive as problems that make you want to overeat. At the end of the week, total the number of days during the week each item was a problem.	M	T	W	T	F	S	S	TOTAL
1. Snacks								
2. High Fat								
3. Sugar								
4. Fast Food Establishments								
5. Troublesome Foods								
6. Eat Until Full or Overfull								
7. Candy								
8. Coffee								
9. Non-diet Cola Drinks								
10. Alcohol								
11. Doughnuts								
12. Salad Dressings								
13. Lack of Home Support								
14. Restaurants								
15. Big Meals								
16. Unaware of Food Consumption								
17. Too Much Red Meat								
18. Craving Certain Food								
19. Social Events								
20. Desserts								
21. No Exercise								
22. Lack of Friendly Support								
23. Lack of Motivation								

Now rank the three problems that you feel are contributing most to your tendency to overeat.

1. ______________________________
2. ______________________________
3. ______________________________

Your 8-Step Personal Action Plan

Each week you will design your own individual Personal Action Plan. This plan, designed by you, consists of weight loss goals and strategies for the next week.

1. Weigh yourself and plot your weight on the Weight Loss Profile Sheet (p. 158).
2. Review your Eating and Exercise Diary and Problem Inventory for the week. Identify any problem eating behaviors that need to be corrected.
3. Select one problem eating behavior and describe it in this week's Personal Action Plan (as shown on the following page).
4. Write down several strategies that you could use to alter this selected problem eating behavior. From these strategies, select a best strategy as a solution and include this strategy in next week's Eating and Exercise Diary. Write the strategy in the space provided at the top of next week's Eating and Exercise Diary.
5. Consult with your partner in planning your complete program for the next week.
6. Plan your daily meal and exercise schedules for next week.
7. Indicate your commitment to the weekly Plan of Action by writing a personal statement of commitment.
8. Develop appropriate rewards for successful completion of the selected strategy.

Self-Understanding Exercises

Setting Goals for Permanent Weight Control

Reflect back on you experience in this program. You have probably learned a lot about yourself and your eating behaviors. Completing the following open-ended statements will aid you in applying what you have learned to your future and your continued success in permanent weight control.

1. The responsibility of checking my eating behaviors will rest almost entirely on ______
   ____

   The way I feel about this is ______________________________

2. The factor that will continue to motivate me to control my weight is ______________
   ____

3. The eating behavior I have most successfully developed on this program is ________
   ____

4. The eating behavior I will continue to reinforce is ______________________________
   ____

5. When I am in social situations I plan to ______________________________
   so I can control my behavior and my weight.

6. The most important thing I learned from being on this program is ______________
   ____

7. The best thing I appreciate about my new self-image is______________________________
   ____

8. In one year from now I can see myself ______________________________
   in terms of my weight control/appearance.

9. In five years from now I see myself______________________________
   in terms of my weight control/appearance.

Exercise for Fat Loss

During the past twenty years, Americans have become more weight conscious with each passing year. Thinness has become the vogue among both sexes and all ages. Numerous research projects have revealed the strong correlation between excess weight and premature death. Unfortunately, the relationship between being overweight and premature overweightness is specifically due to excess fat. A person can appear very thin but may have a percentage of body fat that is very high.

If your overweight condition is attributed to increased muscle mass, the overweight condition should not be assessed as an increased health risk. In most instances excess muscle mass would even be considered a health benefit. There are many examples of obese individuals in our society who actualy are underweight according to acceptable height weight standards. To determine your ideal percent body fat, refer to the Body Fat Classification Chart below:

BODY FAT CLASSIFICATION

CATEGORY	RANGE (%)	
	MEN	WOMEN
Athletic	Less Than 11	Less Than 14
Optimal	11-14	14-17
Acceptable	15-17	18-22
Overfat	18-19	23-27
Obese	20+	28+

To decrease your percent body fat by 1% you will probably have to lose between 1 and 3 pounds of fat. A weight loss program that does not include exercise as a component, is not going to be very effective in helping eliminate fat tissue. If you lose weight but do not reduce your existing percent body fat, it is doubtful that you will have improved your health status. To have your percent body fat assessed, consult with your physician, an exercise physiologist or various other health care practitioners.

The formation of fat cells is a process that begins very early in life. You will have all of the fat cells you will ever have by the time you reach adulthood. Specifically, you will have developed fat cells while in utero during the last three months of gestation, during your first year of life, and during the growth spurt of adolescence. Once you reach adulthood you simply maintain your existing fat cells.

Some individuals have as many as 250 billion fat cells, whereas others, may have as few as 25 billion fat cells. Obviously, the fewer the number of fat cells, the simpler the task of regulating and controlling the formation of fat tissue. This variability in the number of fat cells in individuals accounts for the individual differences we see in people struggling to control their weight. One person appears to be able to eat anything and never gain a pound; while it seems that someone else simply tastes a dessert and gains several pounds.

The best weight control program is one that combines caloric reduction with an aerobic exercise program and a system for changing poor eating habits. **The establishment of a daily exercise routine is especially important if you expect your fat loss to be permanent.** If your lifestyle does not include daily big muscle activity, muscle mass will eventually atrophy into fatty deposits throughout the body. Exercise also provides a tremendous advantage in helping you control your appetite.

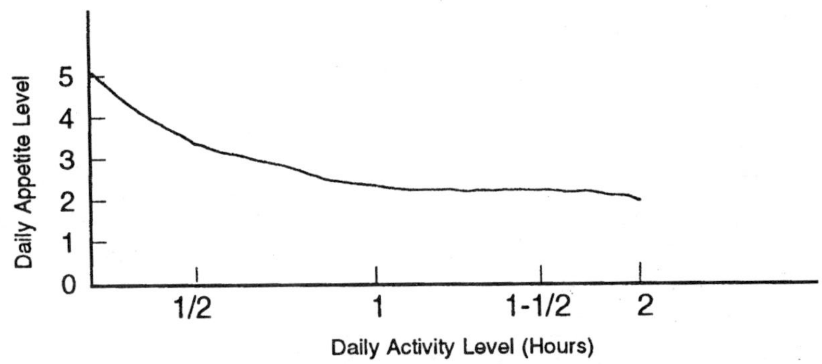

Effect of Exercise on Appetite

All of us generally value the idea that exercise is good for us and important to our well-being. Why is it then that only a small percentage of us engage in regular daily exercise? The excuses developed in the minds of men and women are too numerous to mention here, but in general, the majority of these excuses are reflections of our own individual value systems. Either the information presented by health scientists concerning the value of exercise has not been convincing, or Americans have developed a value system that does not place a high priority on physiological wellness.

The orientation by medical practitioners toward the cure of illness with little or no emphasis on the maintenance or improvement of wellness has certainly contributed to the average American's lack of concern about poor cardiovascular health or poor respiratory functioning, that is, until the crisis finally occurs. When the heart attack happens, or the handicapping effects of sedentary living finally develop, the average person thinks, "now is the time to make an adjustment," and everything can be "cured" or put back to normal. The sad fact is that doctors cannot perform such miraculous works.

The sooner a person begins a daily regular exercise program, the better that persons' chances of living a longer, healthier, happier life. Most people would not dare begin the day without brushing their teeth; but, in terms of improved health and well being, and protection against disease and disability, there is no comparison between daily tooth brushing and daily exercise. It is not uncommon to see physical middle age arrive on someone in their mid 20's when that person does not exercise properly. However, there are also those vigorous youngsters in their 60's and beyond who provide us with living proof that daily exercise will postpone physical aging in adulthood and enhance strength and stamina in old age.

It has now been established that sedentary living and inadequate exercise are factors contributing to headache, backache, muscular weakness, chronic fatigue, joint pain and joint injuries, high blood pressure, coronary artery disease, atherosclerosis, and accelerated aging. It appears that with all this information in support of daily exercise, if people really valued their physical health, they would immediately implement the necessary changes into their daily lifestyles.

The fact is that most Americans have their lives primarily controlled by everything around them and they do not have the power or the understanding and discipline to change their daily habits. The average person is simply "too caught up" in those necessary activities of job responsibility, household chores, parental responsibility, etc., to expend the energy necessary to plan and facilitate a personal behavioral change system. This process becomes even more complex with all the time demands including the hustle and bustle of everyday living. If a person is going to be successful with a physical fitness program for self improvement, there are ten principles that should be carefully reviewed and thoroughly understood, otherwise, the attempt at self improvement is probably not going to be worth the effort. A brief review of these principles is as follows:

(1) **The body of knowledge about the advantages of daily physical exercise is motivating and supportive** of your behavioral involvement in a personal exercise program. You can not lose weight and improve fitness by reading about it, but certainly the information can be encouraging. If you attempt to read and learn more about fitness, you will be more likely to remain "fitness conscious" and committed to your personal program.

(2) **An assessment of your daily lifestyle for the purpose of identifying time frames when exercise can be scheduled is an absolute necessity.** Remember, an adequate program will necessitate at least 30 minutes a day for 4-6 workouts each week. The process of planning and scheduling can not be over-emphasized. If your most desirable form of exercise is one that demands the participation of other people, such as tennis or racquetball, this can be an advantage and a disadvantage. If other people are depending on you, you will be less likely to cancel a scheduled workout because something has "come up" that you feel is more important. However, if you do not have alternative exercise routines that can be performed alone, you might sometimes choose not to exercise because of the hassle of havicontact someone else for a match and being confronted with the problem of working out an appropriate time, scheduling a court, etc. It makes no difference at whime of day you choose to exercise, as long as it fits nicely with your daily routine.

(3) **You must value your exercise program as vital and fundamental to daily living.** The time spent each day must be viewed as something special you do for yourself. If the daily schedule has to be altered, be certain that you are not the one who will be cheated because of too many other things being dumped into the day's activities. Do not let your environment, including other people, control your quest for obtaining and maintaining good health.

(4) **Review all of the various exercise programs and identify the types of activities that are most appealing to you personally.** If you do not enjoy or learn to

enjoy the exercise programs you attempt, you are not likely to continue with the program. There must be pleasurable advantages in conjunction with health advantages or else the activity is not suitable as a unit in a lifetime fitness program. If the program is too expensive, or seasonal, the activity may be inconsistent with the lifetime fitness concept.

(5) **Select activities that can be performed with easily accessible facilities.** Activities such as walking and jogging have widespread popularity because they involve minimal facilities and programs can easily be planned according to individual capability. If you have fitness centers, tennis courts, racquetball facilities, or golf courses, available in you community, these are important considerations in planning your total program. It is generally a good idea to rely on two or three different exercise programs to provide variety and eliminate sameness or routine from your daily schedule. An alternating program of walking, playing tennis, andusing a home rebounding unit would be an example of an excellent combined program. Remember, the exercise programs you select should provide you with some form of exercise for each season of the year. Lifetime, daily fitness should be the major objective motivating your participation.

(6) **Purchase appropriate equipment to minimize chances of injury.** Always wear clothing suitable and appropriate for the environment; be certain to dress warmly if the program involves outdoor activity during the winter. The importance of a stocking cap cannot be overemphasized in extremely cold environments where jogging or intense exercise of some form is being performed. Fifty percent of the body warmth can be lost through the head and neck during exercise. Of all the equipment you will need, if the activity is largely a lower body exercise, proper shoes will be the most important piece of equipment you will purchase.

(7) **Progress slowly in your exercise program.** It may even be advisable to begin your program with a day of rest between exercise bouts. Always do the proper warm-up and cool-down program as this will help eliminate soreness. Attempting to progress too rapidly can result in discouragement and injury. Advancing too rapidly is the major cause of people dropping out of progressive exercise programs.

(8) **Include your spouse or friends in your daily exercise.** If you surround yourself with the right people, frequently the social interaction will become a strong motivating factor to keep you excited about your exercise program.

(9) **Plan your daily schedule to include your exercise program.** The importance of planning cannot be over-emphasized. Establish some relarity to your workouts; this maou of the decision of when, where, and how get your daily exercise.

(10) **Establish short-term and long-term goals including an appropriate reward system for successfully accomplishing these goals.** If you are going to be successful in changing your sedentary life to an active one, you must first identify your goals. The goal setting process must be reasonable and consistent with your physical capabilities and your present level of fitness. If you set your goals too high, you may become easily discouraged and quit. Secondly, you must evaluate your present lifestyle and determine those factors that would most likely

motivate you to accomplish your goals(s). It is very important to state your goals in writing. A special form will be provided in this manual to help you as you prepare yourself for your new exercise program.

The most difficult aspect of changing one's habits involves **MOTIVATION.** People are motivated to exercise by many different factors. Some people are motivated internally, because of physiological problems such as being overweight, feeling sluggish, or a poor self concept. Others are more moticated by external factors, such as wanting to look good for a husband, being able to wear a bikini swimsuit, or it might just be someone saying, "You look nice today." In the early stages of this program, it will be very important to have as much external motivating support as possible. This program has been designed to provide you with much of this support with data recording, contracts, etc. It will be your responsibility to utilize these materials in addition to the establishment of any other personal support that you might be able to gain. It will be your task to assess your own lifestyle to identify "how you are best motivated," and then plug these motivational keys into the reward system of this exercise program. The appropriate data collecting forms will be provided in this text. It is important for you to utilize these materials as a resource in recording your progress and planning your daily exercises while you move through our eight-week plan. It has been our experience that both the record keeping and data review are important factors contributing to your success with this program.

After reading this text, **DO NOT LAY IT ASIDE AND STRIKE OUT ON YOUR OWN, CONFIDENT THAT YOU KNOW ALL YOU NEED TO KNOW TO ESTABLISH YOUR PROGRAM.**

This text will be your guide. Your commitment to use it as recommended will be an indicator of how much success you will have with this program.

Establishing a daily exercise program is difficult to impossible for some people. Reasons for not participating in daily exercise include "it is inconvenient," "I have no place to exercise," "I am too tired," "there is no time in my daily schedule," and "I don't really need muscles anyway." Interestingly enough, these same people who make these excuses, usually do not know why exercise is so important. In the next section we will look at the very personal reasons why everyone needs daily regular exercise.

How to Exercise Safely

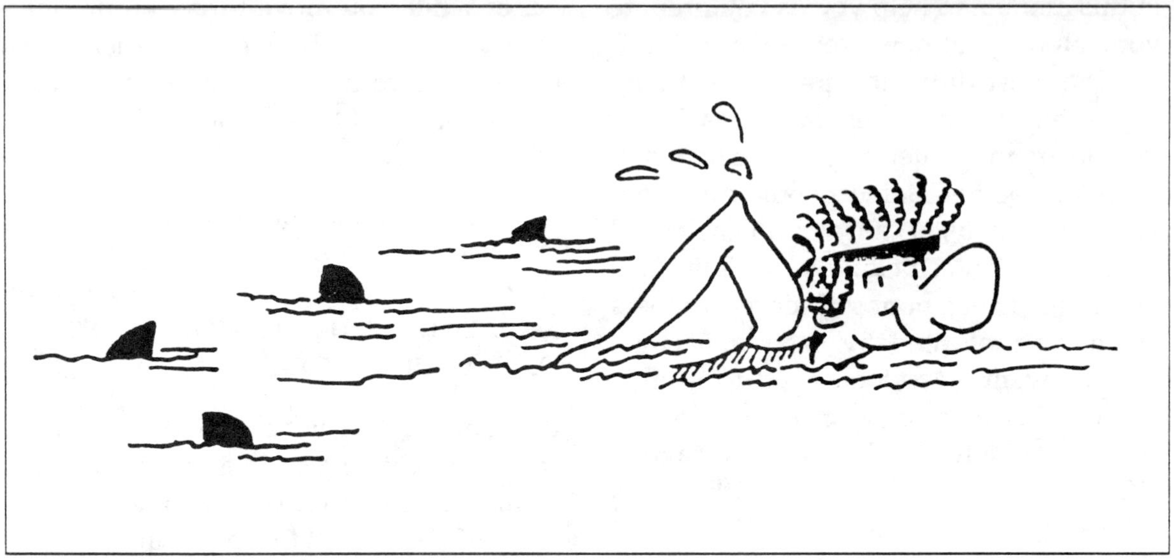

The question of safety in an exercise program is one which should be thought about by anyone interested in becoming physically fit. Usually as one gets older, concern about the safety of an exercise program increases. Many people want to know if the benefits of exercise apply to all ages, and if it is safe to pursue those benefits at all ages.

Safety After Forty

Or after fifty, or after sixty, or after seventy! Is it possible? The aging process in this country is usually associated with a decrease in physical abilities. There is a loss of mobility due to decreases in strength and flexibility. There is a decrease in ability to carry out physical tasks, due to our body's decreasing ability to take in and deliver oxygen. And perhaps worst of all, there is a decreased quality of life due to sickness, disease, and lost mobility. We know these things occur with old age, because we see them all around us. But are these things necessary? Do they have to occur? In the United States, with our reliance on technology for the so-called easier, better life, we become less active and less physically fit as we mature. But do we exercise less because our bodies are less capable of performing, or are our bodies less capable because we do so much less exercise? Since Americans have it so easy, with automation and an abundance of food, we do not really know what potential we have for quality living in the "mature" years.

Scientific studies have proven that age does not affect the fitness benefits of an exercise program. Muscle from a 65-year-old person burns just as many calories and may function just as efficiently as muscle from a 21-year-old individual. People of any age can improve their health and fitness through the **proper** exercise program. An older person may never be totally like a 20-year old, but the sixty-year old can possess excellent health and a zest for life (and maybe be more physically fit than **some** 20-year olds!). This "proper" exercise program is different for each individual, and will probably be different for the same individual at different ages. Before beginning the program, the first consideration is being certain about your ability to become safely involved in a vigorous exercise program.

Visiting Your Doctor

A question of whether or not you need to see your doctor, before initiating a program, is a primary consideration. To answer this question, guidelines have been established by the American College of Sports Medicine (ACSM), a high-respected organization of doctors, physiologists, physical educators, and exercise experts. Their first recommendation reflects an attitude of conservatism; "If you have not had a medical examination in the last two years, see your doctor before starting your exercise program." If you have seen your doctor in the last two years, the ACSM has established other recommendations concerning the possible need for a return visit before starting your program.

If you are under 35-years of age, have no history of heart or blood vessel disease, and you have none of the *primary* risk factors for heart disease, such a cigarette smoking, high blood fats, and high blood pressure, you can enter an exercise program without further medical clearance. If your blood pressure exceeds 140/90 for *either* the top or bottom number, be certain to see your doctor. The ACSM also lists as *secondary* risk factors a family history of heart disease, obesity, and diabetes. If you possess any of these factors, you should consider a conversation with your physician concerning your exercise capability.

All persons over the age of 35 should have a medical clearance before entering their exercise program. There can be no harm in playing it safe. Even if you think these guidelines do not apply to you, you will probably feel better by getting a medical opinion.

To summarize, you should see your doctor if you are over 35 years of age, or if you have not been examined by a physician in the last 2 years. You should visit your doctor nomatter what your age, if you have a personal history of heart or blood vessel disease, or if you have any of the primary risk factors for heart disease.If you have any combination of secondary risk factors, you should at least talk to your personal physician.

Staying Safe Once the Program has Started

What your exercise program consists of will depend on your general health and fitness in the beginning. Once you have received the doctor's OK, the safety of the program depends on the proper type and progression of exercises. If the exercises are chosen properly, and you start easily and build up slowly, there should be no danger involved. Exactly how to safely partici in exercise will be discussed in the next section of this text.

Stay in the Daily Exercise Session

The most hazardous time in an exercise session is the first 10 minutes; your body should be gradually warmed up to your planned activity. Stretching and flexibility exercises are an excellent way to warm up prior to your involvement in more intense exercise. If your exercise session will involvtriding (walking, jogging), the last part of the warm-up should be easy striding. If your exercise session will include strength exercises, the last part of the warm-up should be easy strengthening activity.

The cool-down is equally as important as the warm-up. A proper cool-down will also last approximately 10 minutes. If performed correctly, the cool-down allows time for the heart rate and body temperature to gradually return to normal. An important aspect of the first 3-5 minutes of cool-down is continuous, slow movement. Walking or easy stretching is more gentle and less stressful to the systems of the body than simply coming to a complete stop. More stretching and flexibility exercises allow for further cooling, as well as helping prevent future soreness and injury.

If you are concerned about safety, *always* allow time for warm-up and cool-down. People who have sustained injury or damage from exercise usually have not followed the recommended guidelines, regarding the proper technique for the warm-up and cool-down. You will enjoy your exercise more and receive more fitness advantages if you pay heed to warm-up and cool-down as fundamental components to any form of physical activity.

PHYSICAL ACTIVITY DO'S

1. Establish a new mental outlook on being physically active. Think in terms of using energy rather than saving energy.
2. Use stairs instead of elevators.
3. Increase the amount of walking you do daily by:
   - walking to work
   - parking your car further from your destination
   - getting off the bus several stops earlier
   - doing your own errands; don't send the children
   - doing enjoyable walking (e.g., in the park, hiking, etc.)
4. Avoid buying unnecessary convenience items that save steps.
5. Plan enjoyable group activities into your life on a regular basis (e.g., join a volley ball or bowling team)
6. Get the whole family involved in being active.
7. Check with your physician before making any substantial increase in physical activity.
8. Increase physical activity gradually and on a regular basis.
9. Check out carefully any exercise equipment or establishment before purchase or enrollment.
10. Plan time into your daily routine for enjoyable physical activity.
11. Reward yourself for following the procedures advocated in this program.

PHYSICAL ACTIVITY DON'TS

1. Begin an activity program without yourphysician's consent.
2. Try to do too much too soon.
3. Rely totally on calisthenics. For most people they become boring.
4. Buy convenience items just because they save you steps.
5. Think of physical activity as effort. Think of it as fun.
6. Spend any more time than is necessary sitting.
7. Use your car any more than is necessary.

Why Exercise is Important

Everyone, regardless of age, sex, or physical limitations, needs a minimum of thirty minutes of big muscle activity daily. Thirty minutes of daily exercise should be the minimum standard and should have a higher priority than brushing your teeth each morning.

The advantages of exercise have been carefully researched by medical experts and health professionals. An increasing opinion among health authorities is that if one examines all of the known therapies utilized by physicians to treat illness and promote health, none of these can approximate the total benefits that can be achieved by correctly prescribing regular progressive exercise programs for patients. Exercise has probably contributed more to making sick people well, lame people active, and mentally distraught people enthusiastic and excited about what life is all about than any other therapy available in medicine. This is not to say that exercise is a panacea or a cure-all, certainly that is not the case. All of the recognized, legitimate, therapeutic approaches in medicine should be respected. The problem is simply that the miraculous advantages of exercise have historically been overlooked by many practitioners of the medical arts.

Through research, a powerful body of knowledge concerning the advantages of exercise has now been developed. One of the most significant discoveries is that there now exists a very strong case that exercise may reduce the risk of heart disease. Inone of the first studies to shed light on this relationship, (Zukel, Lewis, Enterline), 1 hour of daily heavy activity lowered the incidence of heart disease to less than 20% of the inactive group. Several other studies have been conducted to help substantiate that exercise does reduce one's risk of heart attack, and although the evidence is inconclusive, the data suggest that exercise probably does provide this important advantage.

It is well documented that physically active individuals have a much better chance of surviving a heart attack than someone who is inactive. Physical activity aids your body in developing additional colateral blood vessels in the heart, thereby improving circulation capabilities and resistance to circulatory disorders.

Circulation is also enhanced in the extremities as well as all vital organ systems. This improves cellular functions and tunes up important digestive, respiratory, excretory, and reproductive systems. Oxygen supply is improved to all cells and organs of the body. A great amount of oxygen carrying blood is supplied to the brain helping you to be more alert mentally. Fats such as cholesterol and triglycerides in the blood stream will be decreased when one exercises properly, reducing the ate of plaque formation in the arteries. This plaque formation is a process that restricts circulation and presently causes more death and disability than any other medical problem. In the person who exercises daily, the arteries will remain elastic and young, the blood pressure will be lower, blood clots will not form as readily, and plaque will develop at a much slower rate.

The total blood volume of a person physically fit will sometimes be increased by as much as a quart, providing you with greater stamina for daily activities or work and play. You will recover more quickly fromfatigue, experience fewer infections, digest your food better, and sleep more soundly. Many people depend heavily on exercise to help maintain bowel regularity and keep all of their body functions at top efficiency. It is an established fact that exercise will speed up one's recovery from illness and/or injury.

In the past ten years mental health therapists have begun to realize the significance of the fact, "you cannot separate the mind and the body." Exercise and recreational activities have become important tools for the practicing therapist. Coincidentally, thousands of anxious, frustrated Americans have begun to recognize the therapeutic advantages of 30 minutes of exercise in their daily lives. Exercise will, unequivocably, enable you to better adapt to and cope with the stresses of life. Daily activity is unequalled in its capacity to help fight or control depression, relieve tension, and give you a fresh relaxed attitude toward the rigors of everyday living.

Further advantages of regular progressive exercise include the maintenance of important muscle tone throughout your body, thereby increasing the rate at which your body burns calories. The active adult or child is not likely to have weight control problems. Exercise will regulate the appestat of the hypothalmus, thereby regulating overeating and body weight. Posture will be improved, and for children, risks of developmental problems associated with bone and muscle development will be lessened. For adults, the aging process is diminished and degenerative conditions are frequently delayed.

A balanced program of exercises utilizing large skeletal muscles in all parts of the body is recommended. Muscles of the extremities, abdomen, back, stomach, and neck should be involved. Strong stomach muscles can help prevent and correct the development of a "pot belly" in your adult life. Strong abdominal muscles and back muscles are also important for the prevention of backaches and shoulder problems characteristic of middle age. A vigorous aerobic program combined with selected stationary exercises appears to be ideal to stretch and contract all the major muscle groups, joints, and ligaments. This type of combined program affords you the best chance of reaping the multitude of advantages associated with exercise discussed in this section.

WHAT EXERCISE WILL DO FOR ME

1. Strengthen the Heart Muscle
2. Increase Production of Red Bllod Cells
3. Lower Blood Pressure
4. Increase Blood Volume
5. Lessen Severity of a Heart Attack Should One Occur
6. Increase Stroke Volume of the Heart
7. Produce a Lower Resting Pulse
8. Eliminate Fat Tissue
9. Improve Lung Capacity
10 Improve Digestion
11. Increase Size, Strength, and Endurance of Muscles
12. Assist in Adapting to Stress
13. Decrease Cholesterol and Triglyceride Levels of the Blood
14. Imrpove Physical Appearance
15. Depress Hunger
16. Decrease Glucose Intolerance
17. Decrease Blood Clotting
18. Promote Bowel Regularity
19. Speed Recovery from Sickness
20. Control Depression
21. Diminish the Aging Process
22. Alleviate Painful Menstrual Cramps
23. Diminish the Number of Infections
24. Increase the Production of Endorphin
25. Assist in Sleeping More Soundly
26. Keep Organ Systems Functioning at their Peak
27. Increase the Size of Blood Vessels

How Exercise Can Help Specific Health Problems

Problem	Foods to Avoid	Types of Exercise
1. Back, knee, or joint problems	If problems are arthritic, avoid alcohol, beer, organ meats of all typs. Control your consumption of salt and sugar. Eat fresh fruits and vegetables. Drink plenty of fluids.	Exercises that do not produce poundingor jolting effects on the joints such as swimming and stationary calesthenics would be advisable. A rebounding aerobics program is preferred.
2. Hypertension (High Blood Pressure)	*Avoid high salt intake including such foods as pickles, condiments, snack foods, and salted meats of all types. The specific diet should be prescribed by a physician.	Regular progressive daily exercise is recommended. An aerobic program of daily walking, swimming, cycling, or rebounding will do much to help lower your blood pressure. Avoid strenuous arm exercises, even pushups and pullups.
3. Circulatory Disorders include Heart Disease and Stroke	Avoid saturated animal fats in such foods as pork, beef, and lamb. Butter, whole milk, and eggs should be limited. High salt foods, sugary foods, shellfish, and organ meats should be eliminated if possible.	Regular progressive exercise (aerobic in nature) should be planned for each day. Exercise will strengthen the heart muscle, build extra blood vessels, lower blood pressure, and help clear clogged arteries.
4. Diabetes	•Candy and sweets of all types. (See your physician for a special dietary plan).	Aerobic exercise such as walking jogging, swimming, rebounding, cycling will help solve the problem of weight reduction and can improve glucose tolerance.

These recommendations are intended as supplements to diet and drug regimens prescribed by your physician.

Adapted from Jean Mayer "Exercise," *Family Health,* February, 1975.

What It Means to be Physically Fit

Being physically fit can mean many things, but generally it means being able to function at top efficiency in your daily activities. We usually think that athletes are physically fit, and most athletes are at a level of good to excellent fitness. However, there are many different aspects of physical fitness; strength, flexibility, coordination, endurance, and percent body fat. Certain sports place unusual demands on our bodies, for example, football players have to be strong, but do not have to possess a lot of endurance. Marathon runners do not have to be able to lift heavy weights, but should be able to keep running for long periods of time.

The important question the average person needs to answer is "do I need to be an athlete to be physically fit?" The answer is absolutely NO, you do not need all of the strength of a football player or the endurance of a marathon runner. You *do* need some of the attributes which these different athletes possess. In order to have total physical fitness, you need to include some form of activity to help develop strength, flexibility, endurance, and promote reduced body fat. Your reasons for trying to become physically fit should be quite different from the athlete whose primary objective is performance while your major objective is improved health. Your choice of exercise and your choice of how much time you spend on that exercise will be decisions based on how much you need exercise to develop, improve, or sustain good health.

There are three types of physical fitness programs that you need to concentrate upon; there are programs that will emphasize aerobics, other programs will be primarily strength oriented and still others will be based largely on flexibility needs. We will discuss each of these, beginning with aerobics, the program that will do most to improve your overall health.

Aerobic Programs

The term "aerobic" means "with air" or "with oxygen." All of the body's processes require oxygen to be completed, including the production of energy for living, moving, working, playing, and exercising. An activity that allows you to bring in enough oxygen to power the energy systems during activity, in effect creating a balance between energy brought in and energy needed, is called an aerobic activity.

The cells of the body have a certain amount of stored energy, a factor that allows our muscles to function effectively for short episodes of activity. The oxygen expended must be put back into the body to repay the debt (called the oxygen debt). These types of activities are called "anaerobic," meaning "without air." Sprinting fast, or climbing a flight of stairs fast, are anaerobic activities, and we breathe heavily after participation in these activities to repay the oxygen debt.

Aerobic activities are by far the most important type of exercise for the average person. Aerobic activities stimulate the most important systems in the body for the maintenance of good health, specifically the heart and the lungs. Circulatory disfunction with heart disease is responsible for the majority of deaths and disabilities in this country. Improvement in the health of the heart and lungs, the systems which take in and deliver oxygen to the body, helps to prevent or delay the onset of heart disease. Furthermore, aerobic activities allow you to burn more calories and control weight better thanother types of exercise programs (we will discuss the advantages of exercise and fat loss in a later section).

Aerobic activities are better for you than anaerobic activities. In fact, anaerobic activities may be dangerous. Anaerobic activities frequently elevate heart rates and breathing rates higher than aerobic activities because they are very intense activities that place unreasonable demands on the body. The high intensity of anaerobic exercise prevents the participant from enjoying enough actual exercise time to stimulate improved functioning of the heart and lungs or burn excess calories; and, maybe more importantly, the short and intense bursts of activity are usually not very pleasant. Therefore, we hope to discourage you from anaerobic exercises and encourage you to participate in aerobic forms of activity. The best way to distinguish between aerobic and anaerobic activity is by monitoring your pulse rate. If you follow the guidelines we recommend, you will have no trouble selecting an aerobic exercise program appropriate

Activities That May Produce Aerobic Training Benefits

• Walking	• Rope Skipping	• Squash
• Jogging	• Cross Country Skiing	• Basketball
• Rebounding	• Downhill Skiing	• Fencing
• Cycling	• Racquetball	• Golf
• Soccer	• Dancing	• Volleyball
• Rowing	• Handball	• Skating
• Swimming	• Tennis	

Strength Programs

We all know that strength is the ability of the muscles to lift weight or overcome resistance. Strength is an important component of fitness for health. We do not mean that you need to develop big, bulky muscles or participate in heavy training for weight lifting contests. Strength training for health purposes increases muscle tone so you will have better posture and be able to carry out your daily activities without undue fatigue. An increased amount of usable muscle tissue burns more calories than fat tissue, even at rest!

All of the major muscle groups in the body should have some type of daily strengthening exercise. Some muscle groups can maintain a healthy level of strength simply due to your daily activities of work and play, other muscles are dependent upon specific exercises that must be performed specifically for the exercise advantages to that muscle group. Most of us do some walking each day, or if we are starting an exercise program, we probably will choose an activity in which we use our legs, such as jogging or bicycling. These activities will keep the legs strong if done regularly. The muscle groups in the upper body, the stomach, chest, shoulders, back and arms, need to be emphasized in a strength program in combination with lower body exercise.

When you begin to plan your physical fitness program, the strength of the stomach and abdominal muscles should be your first priority. A lack of strength in these muscles, combined with poor flaxibility, contributes to chronic low back pain. Millions of dollars are lost each year in industry because of lost work time from low back problems. Many major corporations have found it cheaper to build and staff a rehabilitation center for low back problems than to have the continuing loss of work time. The prescribed rehabilitation program for those suffering from low back difficulties usually consists of increased stomach and abdominal strength building activities and increased utilization of flexibility exercises. It is important to establish a personal program of exercise to include these exercises as a means of prevention of most forms of chronic low back pain.

There are many different ways of exercising muscles to increase strength; muscles can be worked with *isometrics* or *isotonics*. In isotonic work, the muscle can overcome the resistance or weight, and will allow the body to move all the way through the motion. An example would be picking up a glass of water and raising it to the mouth; the arm muscles overcome the weight of the glass and allow the arm to move all the way to the mouth. In isometric work, the muscle can overcome the resistance or weight, and will allow the body to move all the way through the motion. An example would be picking up a glass of water and raising it to the mouth; the arm muscles overcome the weight of the glass and allow the arm to move all the way to the mouth. In isometric work, the resistance or weight is so great that the muscles cannot move it, no matter how hard they work. There is no movement of the body. If someone glued a glass of water to the table, we could not pick it up to the mouth. When a person performs isometric exercise, they are usually straining so hard that they actually stop the flow of blood to the muscle, creating a high pressure "back up" at the heart. This means that the heart has to work extra hard, and creates an unnecessary and potentially dangerous situation. During isotonic exercise, blood flows easily and fluidly, alowing the heart to work more efficiently and safely. Therefore, we will recommend certain isotonic exercises for your exercise program.

Flexibility Programs

Flexibility is defined as the amount of motion available to us at any joint in the body, such as the waist or hip. The amount of flexibility in your body is determined by the muscles, tendons, ligaments, and bones which surround and make up your joints. The tighter and shorter the muscles, tendons, and ligaments, the less flexibility you will experience.

If you lack flexibility, you will not be able to move fluidly through the range of motion at a joint, and this inability can lead to minor aches and pains, injury, and disability. When we assess flexibility as it relates to your health, there are certain areas of the body more important than others. The backs of the legs and the lower back are most important because of their relationship with chronic low back pain. A loss of flexibility in the legs and lower back, produced by a shortening and tightening of the muscles and connective tissues, may initiate a "sway back" posture, which does put a great deal of pressure on the spine and vertebra. If you have enough stomach muscle strength to pull the body back in line, this extra abdominal strength might be sufficient to compensate for this lack of flexibility. The problem is that most of us lack stomach strength, unless we perform some exercise especially for the abdominal muscle group. The combination of poor abdominal strength and poor back flexibility, a problem characteristic of most people, makes many of us prime candidates for low back problems.

There are many flexibility exercises that a person can choose. We hope to provide you with a basic program and teach you the proper techniques necessary to perform the exercises. Most of us have been taught to bounce when we do stretching exercises. Scientists have discovered that the body has a "recoil" mechanism which operates during a stretch, causing the muscle attached to connective tissue to try to return to its original length; the harder the bounce, the harder the recoil. This not only does not stretch the muscles, tendons, etc., but it can lead to injury. There is one very important rule for stretching (flexibility) exercises, DO NOT BOUNCE! The proper technique is to stretch to the point of tightness, hold it for 10-20 seconds; repeat the exercise until a total of 40-60 seconds of stretch has been completed. You will discover that each time the exercise is repeated, the stretch extends a little farther. Remember that the flexibility exercises to be described later are "holding" stretches, instead of "bouncing" stretches.

Stretching Considerations for the "Warm Up" and "Cool Down"

HOW TO STRETCH — Stretching is easy to learn, but there is a right and wrong way to stretch. The right way is a relaxed, sustained stretch with your attention focused on the muscles being stretched. The wrong way, unfortunately practiced by many people, is to bounce up and down, or to stretch to the point of pain. These methods can actually do more harm than good.

If you stretch correctly and regularly, you will find that every movement you make becomes easier. It will take time to loosen up tight muscles or muscle groups, but time is quickly forgotten when you start to feel good.

THE EASY STRETCH — When you begin a stretch, spend 10-30 seconds in the easy stretch. No bouncing! Go to the point where you feel a mild tension, and relax as you hold the stretch. The feeling of tension should subside as you hold the position. If it does not, ease off slightly and find a degree of tension that is comfortable. The easy stretch reduces muscular tightness and readies the tissue for the developmental stretch.

THE DEVELOPMENTAL STRETCH — After the easy stretch, move slowly into the developmental stretch. Again, no bouncing. Move a fraction of an inch further until you again feel a mild tension and hold for 10-30 seconds. Be in control. Again, the tension should diminish; if not, ease off slightly. The developmental stretch fine-tunes the muscles and increases flexibility.

BREATHING — Your breathing should be slow, rhythmical and under control. If you are bending forward to do a stretch, exhale as you bend forward and then breathe slowly as you hold the stretch. Do not hold your breath while stretching. If a stretch position inhibits your natural breathing pattern, then you are obviously not relaxed. Just ease up on the stretch so you can breathe naturally.

COUNTING — At first, silently count the seconds for each stretch; this will insure that you hold the proper tension for a long enough time. After a while, you will be stretching by the way it feels without the distraction of counting.

THE STRETCH REFLEX — Your muscles are protected by a mechanism called the stretch reflex. Any time you stretch the muscle fibers too far (either by bouncing or overstretching), a nerve reflex responds by sending a signal to the muscles to contract; this keeps the muscles from being injured. Therefore, when you stretch too far, you tighten the very muscles you are trying to stretch! (You get a similar involuntary muscle reaction when you accidentally touch something hot; before you can think about it, your body quickly moves away from the heat.)

Holding a stretch as far as you can go or bouncing up and down strains the muscles and activates the stretch reflex. These harmful methods cause pain, as well as physical damage, due to the microscopic tearing of muscle.

LIFE STYLE CHANGE FLEXIBILITY PROGRAM

1 Elongation Stretch—Lying on floor on back. Stretch straight out with arms straight over head. Point the toes, and draw in the stomach and abdominal area. Reach with the arms and the legs. Stretching the entire body.

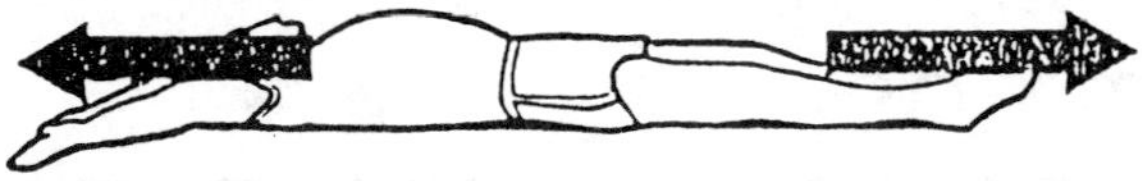

2 Secretary Stretch—Interlace fingers behind head and rest arms on the floor. Now lift the left leg over the right leg. Use the left leg to pull the right leg toward the floor, until you feel a good stretch along the inside of the hip or in the lower back. Keep the upper body flat on the floor. After stretching the right side, cross the right leg over the left and stretch the left side.

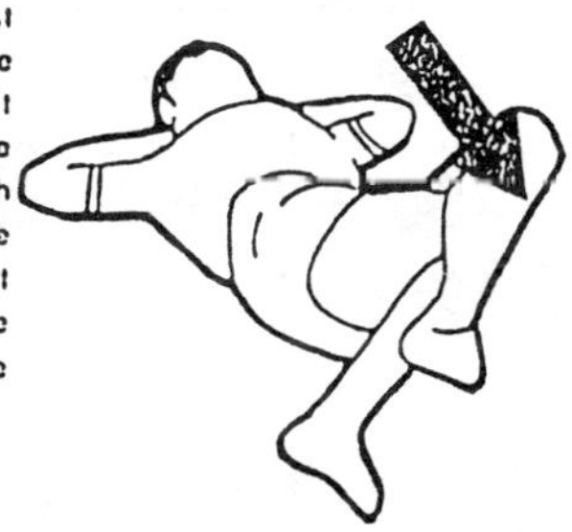

3 Knee to Chest—Lying on floor, pull your right leg toward your chest. Keep the back of your head on the floor. Be sure to keep your lower back flat on the floor. After stretching the buttock area on the right side, lower the right leg down and pull the left leg toward the chest to stretch the left buttock area.

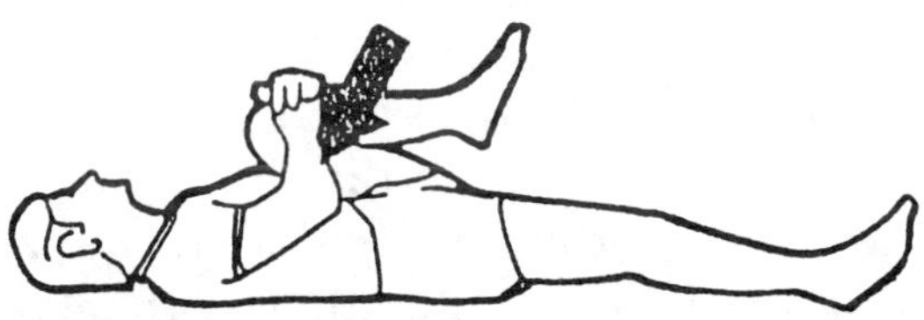

4 Spinal Twist—Sit with your right leg straight. Bend your left leg, cross your left foot over and rest it to the outside of your right knee. Then bend your right elbow and rest it on the outside of your upper left thigh, just above the knee. During this stretch use the elbow to keep this leg stationary with controlled pressure to the inside. With your left hand resting behind you, slowly turn your head to look over your left shoulder, and at the same time rotate your upper body toward your left hand and arm. This should stretch the lower back and side of hip. After stretching in one direction, cross the legs the opposite way and stretch the other direction.

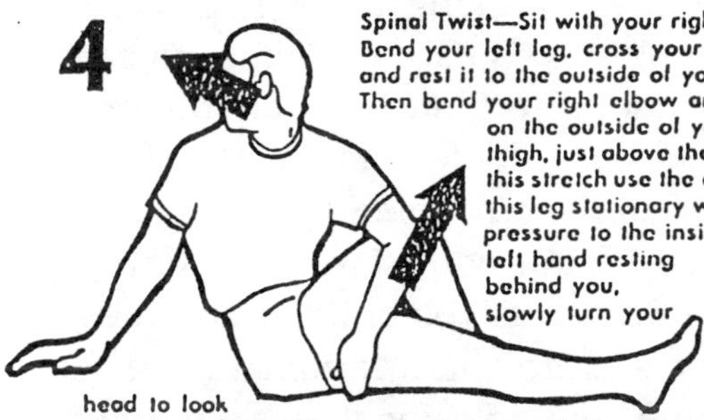

5 Quadricep Stretch—Sit with the right leg bent, with your right heel just to the outside of your right hip. The left leg is bent and the sole of your left foot is next to the inside of your upper right leg. Stretch one frontal thigh area then switch legs and then stretch the other. (You can do this stretch with relaxed leg straight out in front of you).

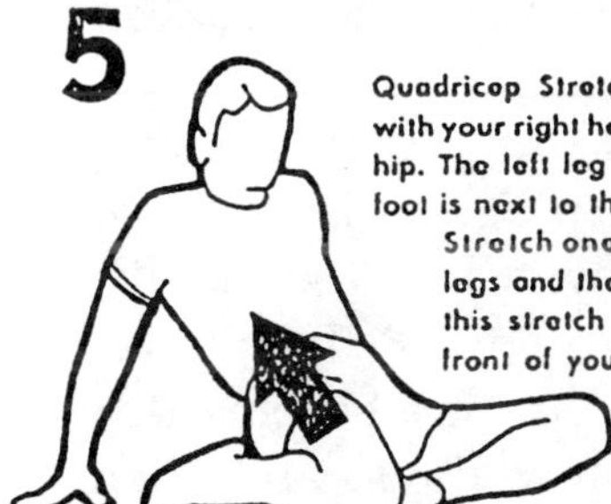

6 Hamstring Stretch—To stretch the hamstring (back of the upper leg), start from the same position as the last stretch except straighten the left leg straight out. Keep the left foot at a 90° angle with the leg. Bend forward from the hips until you feel the slightest stretch, then hold. Concentrate on bending at the hips, not on how far you can reach with the hands. Stretch one leg then the other.

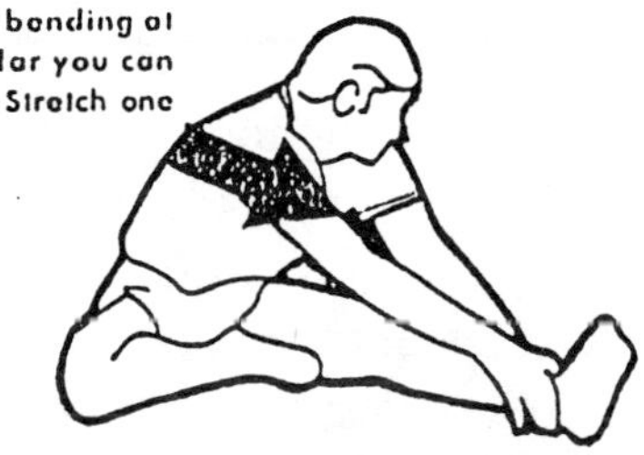

7 Sitting Groin Stretch—Seated on floor, put the soles of your feet together with your hands around your feet and toes. Keep your heels a comfortable distance from your crotch. Now slowly pull your upper body forward, until you feel an easy pull on the inside of the upper thighs. If possible, keep your elbows on the outside of your lower legs. Do not lean from the head and shoulders but bend forward from the hips. Keep your lower back flat and look at a location out in front of you. Do not bounce or jerk the legs up and down.

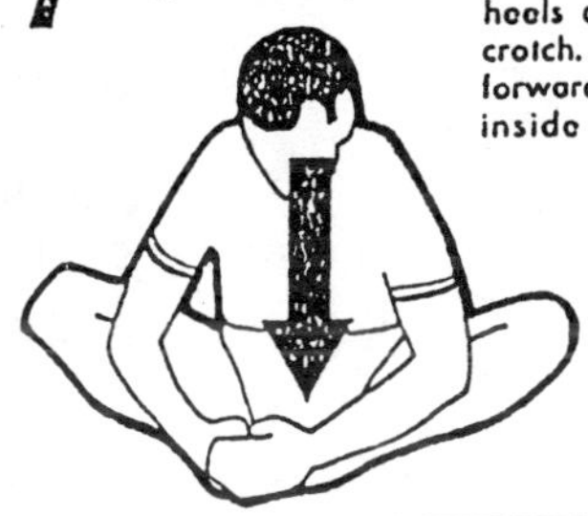

8 Squat Stretch—From a standing position slowly squat down with your feet flat and toes pointed out at about a 20° angle. The closeness of your heels to one another will depend on how limber you are, and what areas you would like to stretch. The squat stretches the front of the lower legs, the knees, back, ankles, achilles, tendon, and deep groin area. Attempt to keep the knees to the outside of your shoulder. The knees should be directly above the toes in the squat position.

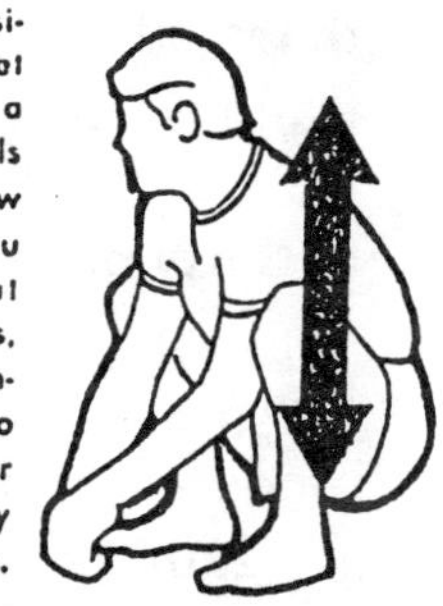

9 Stride Stretch—From a standing position, move one leg forward until the knee of that leg is directly over the ankle. Your other leg goes back to where your other knee is resting on the floor. Now, without changing the position of the knee on the floor or the forward foot, lower the front of your hip downward to create an easy stretch. You should feel this stretch in the front of the hip, hamstrings, and groin. This is a good stretch for lower back problems.

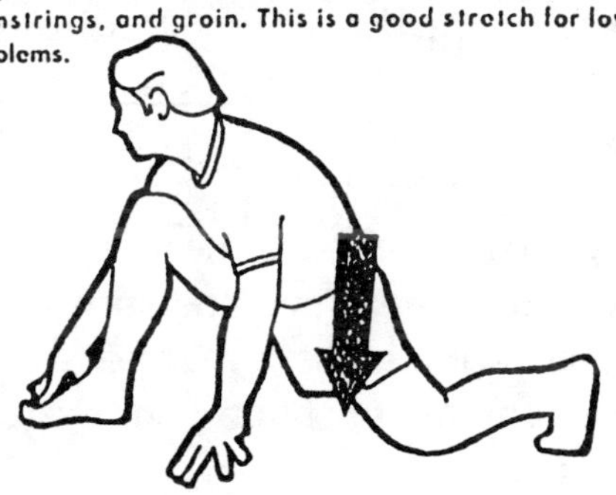

Recommended Aerobic Programs for Fat Loss

Everyone should have some form of aerobic exercise included in their personal fitness program. You should attempt to schedule either striding, swimming, cycling, rebounding, skiing, dancing, racquet sports, or rope skipping into your weekly exercise routine. One or more of these activities scheduled at least 4 times weekly, combined with strength exercises and flexibility exercises will provide you with the esential components for a total exercise program.

Striding

Striding is one of the most natural, healthy forms of exercise. It is an excellent exercise for people of all ages and people with varying levels of physical conditioning. Striding is primarily an exercise for the leg muscles. It is an aerobic exercise that will increase your heart rate to the training level and maintain this elevated heart rate for a duration of at least twenty to thirty minutes.

Depending on your present level of fitness, aerobic striding can range from moderate walking to jogging or running. To gain an aerobic training effect, you must plan to stride briskly enough to raise your heart rate within 60 to 80 percent of its maximum level.

If brisk walking raises your heart rate to produce a training effect, this is the mode of striding you should choose; however, if you find walking is not vigorous enough to elevate your heart rate, you will probably have to increase your tempo to a jog or run. The most important factor in determining the speed of your aerobic stride is the level of exertion you must generate to obtain your target heart rate zone.

To gain aerobic fitness from striding, speed is not the determining factor. Finding your own individualized heart rate target zone and maintaining your stride at this level of intensity is the key to developing a good aerobic striding program. Remember, striding is an individualized program; avoid competing with others when you are walking or jogging. What may be too slow a pace for someone else could be the correct intensity for you.

To gain an aerobic training effect from striding, you should plan to work out a minimum of four non-consecutive days a week. However, as you build your fitness, you may wish to add additional miles to your route, and additional workout days per week. Aerobic fitness will be improved more rapidly if you can schedule a 20 to 30 minute workout, four to six days a week.

The important thing to remember about your aerobic program is that you should learn to enjoy it. Increase the distance and your pace gradually. If you over stress your body, you may become discouraged, skip a few days, and then gradually quit the program totally. A moderate program that you enjoy may motivate you to be consistent and thus help develop an attitude of lifetime aerobic fitness.It may be helpful to remember that the energy expenditure is approximately the same whether you jog or walk. As long as your heart rate is at a training level, yhou will expend almost as many calorics walking a mile briskly as jogging the same distance. Speed is relatively unimportant in terms of calories burned. The important factor to be considered is your heart rate during exercise.

When you begin a striding program, remember that the first six weeks are the most difficult. Your body is adjusting to new demands being placed upon it, and you may experience some soreness and discomfort. To avoid injuries and excessive soreness you should always use the proper warm up and cool down exercises (see pages 120-121). Five to ten minutes is sufficient time to warm your muscles and heart up gradually in preparation for the heavier work load initiated by striding. After your aerobic work out, walking around at a slower pace for approximately five minutes will allow your heart rate and breathing to more gradually return to normal. The cool down exercises are then necessary to lessen soreness and help maintain flexibility of the muscles.

It is a good idea during these intial six weeks to schedule your daily exercise sessions at the same time each day. It is not feasible to presume that you can just incorporate striding into your daily lifestyle. Remember, an aerobic striding program must be maintained at sufficient intensity and for a specific duration of time. Just walking more briskly during your regular daily routine will not satisfy these requirements. By scheduling your daily activities you will begin to develop an exercise habit. Be sure to pick a time that is convenient for you and allows you ample time to do the necessary warm up exercises and the important cool down exercises along with your basic striding program. After six weeks of faithful striding, you will feel so much better, that striding will have become as important to your daily routine as eating and sleeping. You will be surprised to find that your trained body can do more work with less effort and less fatigue. During your usual daily activities, you will begin to experience more energy and tire less easily. At this point, you will be "hooked" on your striding program.You may find that a rigid schedule is no longer necessary as a motivational factor. If you miss one or two days of striding you will not feel quite so well because your body has become accustomed to this healthier style of living.

Striding may produce an even greater improvement in a woman's health than it does for a man. Studies have indicated that striders have significantly better gynecological health. Women striders have easier childbirths, fewer caesarians and fewer miscarriages. Many female striders think menstrual discomforts are lessened by their aerobic activity.

Aerobic striding is a very natural exercise. It does not require special lessons or a specific facility. You can put variety into your exercise by striding in different settings. Even inclement weather is not a deterrent to a strider; if you dress properly, you may find it invigorating to stride in warm weather, brisk cool air, or during a rain shower.

In warm weather you should wear loose fitting, light colored clothing to reflect both the heat and the light. For winter weather, thermal underwear is well designed and comfortable when worn under slacks or under a jogging suit. The extremities, the head and neck should be kept warm, as fifty percent of your body heat can be lost from these unprotected areas. Surprisingly, your striding movement generates enough heat to keep you warm. Do not overdress incold weather. Wear several layers of lightweight clothing that can be taken off as your body warms up. No matter what the weather dictates, the important thing is to dress properly and comfortably for your workout.

If you do not enjoy braving the elements, shopping centers, enclosed malls and gymnasiums provide excellent facilities for striders. These public centers have a controlled year-round environment and offer considerable variety to your daily routine. In many areas, "mall walker" clubs have been formed for the encouragement and social benefits of aerobic striders.

The most important investment a good strider can make is to purchase a good pair of shoes. We have found that a good running shoe also makes an excellent walking and jogging shoe. Aside from your warm-up and cool-down exercises, investment in a good pair of striding shoes is your best insurance against injury. Injured and hurt feet do not produce just a localized pain. When you damage or strain your feet, the pain may transfer to your legs and back. In striding, your feet are the basic weight-bearing foundation. This is why wearing proper shoes is so essential to enjoying your striding program. The shoes you select should have good supports, they should elevate the heel approximately one-half inch above the sole of the foot. The heel should have a cup that firmly embraces the heel and provides strong support. The elevated heel reduces strain on the achilles tendon and protects your foot and ankle from excess strain. A good pair of running shoes should have a thick layered sole running the full length of the shoe and a cushiony inner sole to absorb shock. Flexibility is very important, the shoe should bend easily from heel to toe.

Your big toe should be about a thumbs width away from the end of the shoe. Choose a shoe made of a material that will allow your foot to "breathe"; leather or nylon mesh is usually a good choice.

Finally, be sure to try on both shoes before buying them and check to see if they seem to be a comfortable width. They should be lightweight, yet durable, and your heel should not slide up and down when two pair of socks are worn. After you have purchased your striding shoes, you should wear them only for walking, jogging or running, not for other daily activities.

There are several generalized suggestions that will help you learn to stride correctly. You should stand erect with your back straight but in a naturally comfortable position. Your head should be kept erect with your eyes focused ahead, not on your feet. Your arms should be held comfortably away from your body. When walking, your arms should swing freely at your side. If you are jogging or running, your arms should be bent at the elbows with your hands hanging relaxed from the wrist. Make a special effort to help your shoulders and arms stay relaxed. Occasionally shaking the arms and shoulders may help reduce any tightness that may develop. Your foot should hit the ground heel first, then the body should rock forward so that the weight is transferred to the ball of the foot. If you stride on your toes or with your weight entirely on the balls of your feet, you will increase your chances for shin splints or sore calf muscles.

If you think you are too busy to spare 20 to 30 minutes a day to improve your health, remember that after your first heart attack you will have plenty of time. Striding is an excellent aerobic exercise that takes less time than most forms of aerobic recreation. Like other types of aerobic activities, striding will lower your heart rate, increase your circulation, and decrease your blood pressure. As you begin to "hit your stride" more regularly you will notice a definite psychological advantage. You will be more relaxed during your daily activities, you will work more efficiently and you will sleep better. In adition to being in better physical condition, you will have the extra added bonus of gaining an overall feeling of optimum well being.

Approximate Caloric Expenditure Associated with Various Striding Activities

Calories Activity	Total Speed	Per Minute	Calories Burned
12 minute mile (fast walk)	5 mph	10.0	120
8 minute mile (jogging)	7.5 mph	15.0	120
6 minute mile (running)	10 mph	20.0	120

Summary of Striding Technique

1. Always warm up with a complete stretching program to loosen the muscles and prepare your body for more strenuous exertion.
2. As you begin striding, attempt to hold your head erect while you keep your back straight, and your abdomen as flat as possible.
3. Keep your toes pointing straight ahead and allow your arms to swing freely at your sides.
4. As you stretch forward with your leg, land on your heel and roll your foot forward and push off the ball of your foot. Walking or striding in a flat footed fashion can cause soreness and premature fatigue.
5. Attempt to take long easy strides being careful not to over-exert and pull muscles or ligaments.
6. Breathe rhythmically in full deep breaths (if the temperature is cold, be certain to breathe through the nose and not the mouth as this may be an open invitation to a sore throat.)
7. Cool down with a complete stretching program to help eliminate soreness and tightness.

Swimming

Swimming is rapidly becoming one of the most popular types of exercise for developing total fitness. Thanks to the availability of public indoor pools and the decreased cost of owning your own private pool, many people are gaining more access to swimming as a form of regular daily exercise.

Water exercises can be enjoyed by all age groups and by both healthy and handicapped people. Thanks to the buoyancy associated with swimming, even people with paraplegia, rheumatic heart, emphysema, polio, stoke, and amputation can exercise and enjoy this weightless movement. Swimming is also an excellent therapy for any person with a knee or low back injury. The buoyancy of the water makes it possible to strengthen muscles and joints with relatively little pain.

If you are excessively overweight or have chronic injuries caused by running, or "old football injuries," swimming may be an excellent aerobic exercise for you. Swimming at an aerobic pace with your heart rate at the appropriate target zone produces a training effect for your heart and circulatory system without the stress and strain on your muscles imposed by other aerobic exercises. Swimming enables you to strengthen many of the major muscle groups of the arms, chest, abdomen, back, and legs with the added advantage of having the water to buoy you up, thereby inhibiting the stress imposed on the muscles or joints by gravity.

Water pressure, even on a non-moving person, will stimulate the heart to pump blood throughout the body more rapidly. Swimming activities have been proven to be especially helpful in improving circulatory problems in the arms and legs. Women that have excessive broken vessels in their thighs, have noticed a decrease in the number of these broken vessels after engaging in an aerobic swimming program.

If your swimming program is continuous and rhythmic, it will strengthen your muscles, heart and circulatory system with a very low risk of injury. Few recreational swimmers develop muscle or joint problems provided they abide by a sensible warm-up routine prior to their exercise bouts.

It is just as important for you to utilize the 5 to 10 minute warm-up and cool down exercises as part of an aerobic swimming program as it is for the strider to use this same warm-up program. If you prepare for your aerobic exercise properly, you will lessen your chances for injury and muscle soreness, which as has been mentioned, can be a deterrent to your staying with your exercise program.

Even if you are not an excellent swimmer, you can gain aerobic fitness from swimming, if you will exercise properly. Aerobic swimming is not a competitive sport, you are not judged on your form, style or speed; the only thing you should be concerned about is reaching your target heart zone and sustaining it for 20 to 30 minutes. At the onset, you may find it difficult to sustain your strokes for 20-30 minutes of continuous swimming; however, as you continue to swim on a regular basis, you will grow stronger and your swimming stokes will improve. If your arms become tired, rather than stopping and resting, try slow running back and forth across the shallow end of the pool. The important factor is keeping your pulse rate elevated. do whatever is necessary to keep your body moving. A respectable overhand crawl will not only strengthen you aerobically, but will burn calories at a good rate of about nine per minute.

Much like other aerobic activities, to avoid boredom, you may need to vary your program. Use a variety of strokes and develop several of your own routines. It might be helpful for you to know that the backstroke burns 8 calories per minute, the breast stroke 7 calories per minute, and the more demanding butterfly stroke 12 calories per minute. A thirty minute workout will burn approximately 500 calories, while strengthening the heart, lungs and muscles.

One of the basic strokes that you will probably utilize the most, will be the overhand crawl. If you use the crawl correctly, you will experience less stress on your arms. If you are over 25 years old and did not recently learn to swim, you were probably taught how to do the crawl by the old method of pulling your arm up out of the water, keeping it close to your ear, and pushing it forward with your hand cupped as you cut it back into the water. The newer version of the crawl is easier and less stressful to your arms and shoulders. With this new method, you keep your elbow bent as you bring your arm out of the water and you enter the water again at a point parallel with the midline of your body. Keeping your elbow comfortably bent, pull your whole arm towards your groin. This is a much more natural and less tiring style of stroke. If you learn to master the technique it will make your swimming more enjoyable.

Another suggestion to enhance your swimming experience and add variety to your routine is to use a scuba mask and snorkel. Even though you might think it is a little strange to use this equipment in a swimming pool, the mask will keep water out of your eyes and help prevent eye irritations. The snorkel will solve the problem of breathing and stroking at the same time. While swimming with your head under water, you may enjoy the quiet world you will experience. This may offer you an excellent time to get lost in your thoughts and meditate in the silence of the water. Some people find this to be a much more relaxing way to swim; however, we do not advocate using scuba fins. This usually lightens your workload too much, and lessens the aerobic benefits.

Although swimming activities produce few external injuries, some people who have not swam or exercised vigorously in several years may be vulnerable to shoulder tendonitis. Tendonitis is attributable to the tightening of the tendons associated with age and lack of use. Since our daily jobs and activities do not usually require us to lift our hands over our heads, we lose our flexibility.

Another problem you might develop if you swim regularly is "swimmer's ear." Swimmers' ear is an inflammation of the ear canal caused by the growth of a fungus in a moist, warm, dark place. Being careful to dry your ears and extract all water from the areas may help you avoid this irritation. Ear plugs may be advisable if you are prone to ear infections.

The major investment a swimmer should make is a good comfortable swimming suit that is not designed for fashion but for swimming. It should be made of a nonrestrictive material that allows you to move through the water smoothly. For a woman, the straps of her suit should give her good support but not be restrictive. Usually a one piece is more comfortable for long distance swimming rather than the two piece bikini suits. Many sporting goods shops have a good selection of "swimming" suits that will have the nec essary features to make your aerobic swim more comfortable and enjoyable. Just as a good pair of shoes are of paramount importance to the strider, a good swimming suit is necessary to extract optimal enjoyment and benefit from your swimming program.

CYCLING

"If you are beginning to develop an hour glass figure with all the sand setting in the bottom, cycling might be a good activity to help you redistribute this sand." Cycling is a non-weight bearing exercise that is especially good for the over-weight and the older person. Cycling is not as injury safe as swimming, but a cyclist will experience fewer foot, knee and leg injuries than a strider.

Because of the increasing cost of gasoline, cycling has become not only healthy but practical. Between 1972 and 1976 bicycles outsold automobiles by nearly 10 million units. Even though the cycling boom of the 1970's may be over, a recent government survey ranked cycling second to striding as the country's favorite recreational sport.

Cycling, like other aerobic programs, is an excellent activity to stimulate the heart, lungs and leg muscles. It is also a good exercise to help lose excess pounds and inches. If you ride a bicycle at a moderate pace of six miles per hour on level ground, you will expend 300 calories in an hour. As in striding, cycling primarily exercises the leg muscles, therefore, specific exercises are recommended on pages 45-48 to help strengthen your arms and abdominal muscles.

For many people, cycling is an escape from the pressures and problems of life. Recreational cycling down a country lane or through the early morning streets before the rush hour traffic begins can be very stimulating and relaxing. However, to gain an aerobic training benefit from your riding, there are more important factors to be considered than just the scenery.

You should first choose a relatively flat terrain where you will not need to continually adjust the gears on your bicycle for the hills and valleys. If you will select a flat route for your aerobic cycling program, you can better regulate your heart rate and keep it at the appropriate training level. If you do not have a multi-speed bicycle and your route is frequented by many hills, you may over exert yourself and push your heart rate into the danger zone while climbing the hills. The opposite problem is also presented when you use your multispeed bicycle and gear down too much so that very little effort is exerted to pedal downhill. Your workload will be too light and lessen the aerobic benefits. Therefore, if you choose to ride a multi-geared bicycle, attempt ton minimize as many variables as possible. Select a flat area for your route and make sure you have the gears set correctly so that the activity stimulates your heart enough to reach your exercise target zone. It may take a little practice and experience to determine the appropriate intensity to obtain a training effect, but by checking your pulse rate at 10 minute intervals, and adjusting your gears accordingly, you will soon discover the appropriate level. Remember, the important factor is reaching your target zone heart rate and maintaining this level of stimulation for at least 20 to 30 minutes.

You must plan your aerobic cycling program to meet certain standards of stimulation and duration. Simply deciding to ride your bicycle to work every day may not afford you with sufficient intensity, or a long enough duration to challenge your muscles and heart. Only by monitoring your pulse rate can you determine if your program is providing you with an adequate aerobic workout. If you decide to cycle outdoors, remember to eliminate as many variables as possible. Controlled intensity will enable you to have a constant and rhythmic program that meet the criteria of aerobic exercise.

Using an indoor stationary bicycle or bicycle ergometer helps reduce the variables imposed by the outdoor terrain. However, even with the stationary bicycle, there remains a certain amount of individualized adjustment necessary to achieve an aerobic training benefit. The exercise challenge on the stationary bicycle is not provided by the terrain, speed or gears, but by the resistance knob. Proper adjustment of the stationary cycle is fundamental to a good program.

The more expensive stationary cycles have a more reliable resistance mechanism which is easier to read and regulate on a daily basis. The lesser expensive stationary cycles have a knob which applies resistance as it presses against the front wheel. If there are no measured graduations on the resistance knob, you will have to calibrate your own resistance settings. You may wish to mark the knob once you have found the correct pressure to provide you with enough stimulation to push your heart into your target training zone. With a little patience, you can monitor your pulse rate and adjust the resistance knob until you find the right combinations. It is not advisable to leave your resistance knob set at this pressure when your bicycle is not in use, as this will soon cause variation in the pressure level.

Neither the stationary cycle or the road bicycle is a more preferred means of aerobic cycling. Both methods can provide you with aerobic benefits if you have individualized your program and determine your own personal level of stimulation. Stationary cycling is safer and can be done in the privacy of your own home without weather deterrents or hazards of the open road. If boredom becomes a problem for your stationary cycle program, you might try to cycle while watching television or listening to music. If you decide to initiate an outdoor cycling program, there are a few safety precautions you should consider:

(1) Educate yourself to become a defensive cyclist. Most collisions between cyclists and automobiles are caused by negligence of the cyclist. An estimated one million accidents each year are associated with bicyclists. The U.S. Consumer Product Safety Commission has listed the bicycle as this country's most hazardous product.

(2) Learn bicycling safety, learn the rules of the road, and wear light-colored clothing that can be easily seen. If you must ride in traffic, a florescent bicycle flag mounted on a long pole on your rear wheel or bumper will make you more visible to motorist.

(3) Always wear a bicycle helmet. Statistics show that head injuries account for most fatalities and serious disabilities.

(4) If you need to ride in cold weather, wear layers of loose fitting clothing that will allow you to remove them easily as your body temperature rises., Conversely, riding in hot weather requires light colored clothing and a careful balance of your water intake to avoid overheating and heat exhaustion. If possible, you should avoid riding during daily periods of intense heat and choose a more moderate time to exercise.

Even though stationary and road cyclist seem to be less likely to develop pulled muscles, twisted joints and sore tendons, it is recommended that you warm up properly before beginning your program. Since some cyclist tend to have tight hamstrings and achilles tendons, the general stretching and flexibility exercises in section four will help prevent soreness and injury. In addition, a 5 to 10 minute moderate ride, prior to your aerobic program, will be helpful in warming up your muscles. It is also recommended that you cool down with a similar moderate pace before finishing your workout with various stretching exercises.

Often times, a cyclist will experience knee pain from riding on an improperly adjusted bicycle seat. If the seat is too high or too low, your leg muscles will not be able to function at optimal efficiency. Much of your energy will be wasted working against the bicycle. For proper adjustment, your knee should have a slight bend in it when your foot is on the pedal in the downward position.

Another common complaint of the cyclist is saddle discomfort caused by hard narrow bicycle seats. You may try adjusting the angle of the bicycle seat to lessen the discomfort or, if this is not effective, you may need to try different sizes and styles of saddles until you find the proper fit. If you are suffering from a lot of rubbing and chafing, check your shorts to see if they are too tight or have heavy seams which may be the cause of irritation. Special cycling shorts are available that are made of soft nonrestrictive material with no seams in the crotch.

If you are not accustomed to the traditional tripod position of the bicycle rider you may experience pain in your hands and back. When you ride in the tripod position, keep your weight evenly balanced on your feet, seat, and hands with your back comfortably stretched out over the handlebars. Too much pressure on the hands is not advisable. If you experience a numbness in the little finger and the fourth finger you may need to adjust the height of the handlebars, pad the handlebars, or wear special cycling gloves that are designed to counteract the pressure. If the numbness continues, plan to see your doctor and switch to another type of aerobic activity.

Finally, some cyclist experience low back pain. Stretching out over the handlebars may make you feel awkward and tense. This tension may cause your back, neck, and shoulders to ache. To prevent this type of discomfort, you may need to consciously try to relax more during your ride. If relaxing does not help, you might try adjusting the height of your handlebars and saddle. However, keeping your abdominal muscles strong is your best insurance against low back pain. If you already experience low back problems, you may wish to try alternate types of aerobic exercise. Rebounding or swimming may be a more appropriate exercise for you.

Other Aerobic Activities

We have attempted to provide you with a comprehensive overview of four of the most effective aerobic activities; striding, bicycling, swimming and rebounding. Your primary aerobic program should include one or more of these activities scheduled regularly, however, there are many level two and three aerobic activities you may choose to supplement your total fitness program. It is very important for you to include as much variety as possible if your aerobic fitness program is to become a permanent characteristic of your lifestyle.

It is possible for you to gain an aerobic training benefit from running up and down stairs in your apartment building or home; however, most people would not be motivated to run the stairs for the rest of their lives. Your exercise program should provide you with some aesthetic and recreational advantages in addition to health benefits. If your program is enjoyable, you will be motivated to develop a habit of lifetime fitness. If improving your health is your only motivation, you will most likely become bored and slowly phase the program out of your daily routine.

A list of level one, level two and level three aerobic activities is provided for you on page 124. We have classified many of the level two and level three activities accordingly, because they are limited by the weather, availability of facilities, or the participants skill level. Utilize as much variety of activity as is possible in planning your weekly program. Because of their widespread popularity, we have chosen racket sports, cross country skiing, dancing and rope jumping as level two activities. These activities provide good aerobic benefits and are very attractive social activities enjoyed by many people.

Racket Sports

The term racket sports refers to tennis, racquetball, badminton, and squash. Although these activities utilize different facilities, an appeal to different personalities, they are similar in the demands they place upon the body. All of the racket sports involve rapid twist flexion and extension of the back muscles and sudden bursts of energy from the buttocks muscles, thigh muscles and calf muscles. To be able to participate at a high level of skill, all of your physical and mental energy is required. To discover real pleasure from racket activity you will have to become a student of the sport and learn strategy, scoring, etc. Racket activities require total involvement of mind and body and should become more enjoyable as your skill level improves.

The greatest disadvantage if racket sports is that whenever you have a match, there will always be a winner and a loser. If you cannot keep "winning" in perspective, playing can produce anxiety and stress. Your main purpose of playing will hopefully be to enjoy the stimulating and invigorating benefits of exercise. If you can resolve the competition factor of racket sports, you will enjoy the many benefits associated with this form of exercise.

The aerobic benefits you receive from racket sports, like other activities, are largely dependent upon how often you participate and how hard you participate. If your level of skill is such that you are able to keep the ball going long enough to keep your feet moving and your heart rate in your target zone, racket sports can become a good supplement to your total aerobic program. An analysis of racket sports indicates a rising and failing heart rate among participants due to short bursts of muscular activity followed by briefs periods of rest. You should not make the mistake of depending entirely upon racket sports to provide you with your primary source of aerobic activity. Racket sports are utilized best when combined with level one activities of striding, swimming, rebounding, or cycling.

Cross-Country Skiing

Cross country skiing is preferable to down hill skiing as an aerobic activity. Downhill skiing requires strength, coordination and balance; however, it is difficult to keep your pulse rate elevated and consistent with the inconsistency of the down hill terrain. Downhill skiing, much like racket sports is an activity characterized by short bursts of energy followed by brief periods of rest. The heart rate is difficult to maintain at the target level with the inconsistent workload associated with this type of exercise. Cross-country skiing is gaining popularity because it is more accessible than downhill skiing and provides an aerobic workout similar to striding.

If you are fortunate enough to live in a climate that has a steady snow cover, cross-country skiing would be a good winter activity to augment a stationary cycling or rebounding program. Cross-country skiing is an excellent total body conditioner. The combination of upper and lower body movement provides cross-country skiers with one of the most complete forms of aerobic fitness.

Dancing

One of the newest developments in physical fitness is aerobic dancing. Rhythm and melody are the primary motivational forces for these exercises. The fast pace movements associated with dancing involve a large amount of stretching and flexibility and are a good total body conditioner.

Aerobic dancing can be organized for a social group or as an individual activity in the privacy of your own home. If you enjoy group exercise, be certain to enroll in an aerobic class that is appropriate for your age. This will insure that the pace of the workout is compatible with your own training heart rate.

Aerobic dancing is one of the most effective total body conditioning programs. It is not dependent upon weather or facilities. Aerobic dance can be social without being competitive. If you enjoy music and the relaxation of moving to rhythm, dancing may be your best choice for a good aerobics workout.

Rope Jumping

Watch a winning team after the final point is scored, or a housewife hit the jackpot on a television game show, and you will see a lot of jumping and hopping. Jumping seems to be one of our natural human instincts when under stress. Many housewives, executives, and athletes have discovered that there are outstanding fitness benefits associated with exercise programs that involve jumping.

Rope jumping is one of the least expensive activities which yields the highest aerobic benefits per minute. Ten minutes of rope skipping at a training heart rate level will burn approximately the same number of calories as 30 minutes of jogging at the same heart rate. No special equipment is needed except for a rope of proper length. An ordinary sash cord will suffice, however, you may wish to purchase a manufactured jump rope with ball-bearing handles. Be sure to obtain a rope long enough to reach from armpit to armpit while passing under your feet.

Rope skipping provides an excellent supplementary activity for skiers, tennis players and golfers. Jumping rope strengthens the muscles of the legs, ankles and feet and promotes stronger wrists. A program of rope skipping will improve your balance, agility, and coordination. The rhythmic turning of the rope exercises the upper body as well as the legs. The jumping motion produces an alternating contracting and relaxing motion of the muscles in the legs; this improves muscle tone and speeds the return of the blood to the heart, thus improving circulation.

Since rope jumping is highly demanding (about 3 times more vigorous than jogging), there is a danger of exceeding the training heart rate level. To initiate a rope jumping program, you should probably alternate periods of skipping rope and walking until you can work up to 500 consecutive skips. It is necessary to monitor your heart closely. To prevent rapid increases in your heart rate, you may wish to jump by skipping over the rope one foot at a time.

Rope jumping is a simple, inexpensive, and convenient form of aerobic activity. It is fun, relaxing, and a very natural supplement to other aerobic sports and activities.

How hard you should exercise each time you engage in physical activity is one of the most difficult decisions for the physically unfit individual. How hard to exercise is commonly referred to as "intensity" of exercise. Intensity levels determine whether or not you are receiving a training benefit from your exercise, but more importantly intensity determines whether or not you are exercising safely.

Many of us, particularly those of us who have participated in organized sports, have been taught that we have to pay a price of pain to "get in shape." The old philosophy of "No Pain, No Gain" has been engrained in us through involvement in athletic training programs. As adults, if we decide to try to improve our physical fitness, we frequently revert to the only type of training program with which we are familiar, one that is usually associated with intense pain and periods of severe muscular fatigue.

What is now realized about physical fitness is that athletic training and exercising for health are two distinctly different objectives that are realized through different types of training programs. Exercising for health does not have to be and should not be painful or difficult. There will be some effort and work involved, but never so much as to cause long lasting fatigue or soreness. The best way to prevent negative effects of pain and sore muscles is to regulate the intensity of your exercise and keep it in accordance with your capabilities.

The intensity of your exercise also determines the amount of strain that will be placed on the various systems of you body. When the exercise program is aerobic, the principle organs of concern are the heart and lungs; for strength programs, the muscular system is of major importance; and for stretching or flexibility programs, connective tissue including ligaments and tendons will receive most of the stress bearing responsibility.

Aerobic Programs

We have identified aerobics as being most important for health because of its relationship to this country's most serious degenerative disease, heart disease. The intensity of aerobic exercise correlates with the amount of strain being placed upon the heart. Therefore, the best way of establishing and controling the workload of aerobic exercise is by heart rate. Your heart rate at any given time reflects how hard your heart must work in order for your body to receive the necessary oxygen to function effectively (resting, working, playing, etc.). Everyone should become familiar with their own personal heart rate and understand how their heart rate will change as the work load for their body increases.

FINDING YOUR PULSE—Each beat of the heart pushes blood through the arteries of the body. We can feel the surge of blood if we place our fingertips very carefully on one of these arteries. Each surge of blood will equate to one beat of the heart. You might be able to feel this surge on any artery of the body but there are two places where this pulse can be felt more readily. One of the easier and more accessible sites is the radial artery. The radial pulse can be detected on the underneath side of the wrist on the thumb side. To properly detect the pulse, lay the top side of one wrist into the palm of the other hand. Wrap the fingertips around the wrist, place the tips of the fingers just past the wrist bone. Apply a small amount of pressure, but not so much as to stop the flow of blood. You should be able to feel the pulsations as blood is pumped through the artery.

A second site that might be utilized to find the pulse is the carotid artery. The carotid artery is located on the inside of the neck. To properly detect the carotid pulse, begin by placing the fingertips on the "adams apple," roll your fingertips to the side around the throat and windpipe; you should be able to feel the pulse on the side oh the "adams apple" as your fingers reach the indention of the neck.

The carotid artery has a protective mechanism in it which **lowers** the heart rate when it senses too much pressure. When you check your pulse by feeling the carotid artery, let the artery "jump" to your fingertips instead of applying unnecessary pressure. If you cause the heart rate to go down while taking the pulse, you will not get a true reading of how hard the heart is working.

COUNTING THE PULSE—Heart rates are always expressed as "Beats Per Minute" or BPM. The most accurate heart rate is one which the beats or pulses are counted for one full minute. If you stop to check your pulse during an exercise bout, your heart will immediately begin to slow down. Therefore, the full 1 minute count may not be an accurate indication of how hard your heart is working during exercise. To compensate for this change, you should stop your exercise and immediately count the number of beats in ten seconds and multiply the count by six (to obtain a full one minute count). The chart on the following page shows various ten second counts and the heart rate they represent. To get the ten second interval, you will need to have a watch or clock available that has a sweep second hand or a digital display of seconds. Attempt to take your resting heart rate utilizing this method.

HEART RATES FROM 10-SECOND COUNTS

10-Second Count	HEARTRATE (Beats /per/minute)
9	54
10	60
11	66
12	72
13	78
14	84
15	90
16	96
17	102
18	108
19	114
20	120
21	126
22	132
23	138
24	144
25	150
26	156
27	162
28	168
29	174
30	180

Your pulse should never go above this level.

Some of you feel that you will never be able to locate your pulse and heart rate and count it accurately. Rest assured, it does get easier with practice, and during exercise the pulse will be much stronger. Practice is important if your assessment is to be accurate. If you have difficulty counting your pulse, you may choose to purchase a heart monitor to use during your exercise workout. There are now on the market several pulse monitors that will display your heart rate if you have the sensing device attached to the prescribed part of the body. Monitors can be purchased that will detect the pulse in the hand when you grip the device; some use a fingerclip sensor; some attach to the ear lobe; and still others are wrapped directly around the chest, much like and EKG. For many people, the convenience is worth the expense for a good heart rate monitor.

Heart rate monitors will usually work best if you are motionless. If you stride, rebound, swim, cycle, or jump rope, you should stop to get a true and accurate reading. If the monitor takes longer then 10 seconds to sense and accurately display the pulse, the delay may render the device inappropriate for you workout. Accuracy in assessing your heart rate is of the **utmost** importance; gross inaccuracy resulting from your own inability to count your pulse, or from the inconsistency of an electronic monitor can be dangerous.

WHAT IS THE EXERCISE HEART RATE

How high you allow your heart rate to climb is a measurement of how hard you are working. It is **very** important that you do not overwork yourself. You should always exercise safely and comfortably. The more uncomfortable your exercise, the less likely you will stay with that on a regular basis. Progress in the program is important, but not as important as regularity. Be certain to follow our guidelines for heart rate!

the heart rate at which you exercise, or target heart rate, should reflect your age, capabilities, and current level of fitness. Later you can adjust your target heart rate depending upon your level of fitness; but initially, you should determine your heart rate by your age.

As your age increases, your target heart rate decreases. To determine your target rate subtract your age from 220. Most people should start their program at a target heart rate equal to 60% of the difference between 220 and their age. Therefore, the target heart rate for someone beginning a physical fitness program is:

220 minus your present age x .60

It will be very difficult for you to keep your heart rate exactly on the target during exercise. There is an allowable range, called the target heart rate zone. Your target heart rate will be 5 beats per minute above your target heart rate and 5 beats below your target heart rate.

If you are 40 years of age, your target rate would be computed:

220	Constant
-40	Present age
180	
x .60	Factor for person beginning a program
108	Pulse rate for each minute during your exercise program.

Once your level of physical fitness has improved, after several weeks in your progressive exercise program, you may elevate your heart rate to the 70% level. If you are 40 years of age, your new target heart rate would be computed:

220	Constant
-40	Present age
180	
x .70	Factor for person beginning a program
126	Pulse rate for each minute during your exercise program.

As your fitness level improves, you may eventually raise your training heart rate to the .80 level. There is no reason to ever raise your training heart rate above the .80 level, this will only increase risks without any significant health advantages.

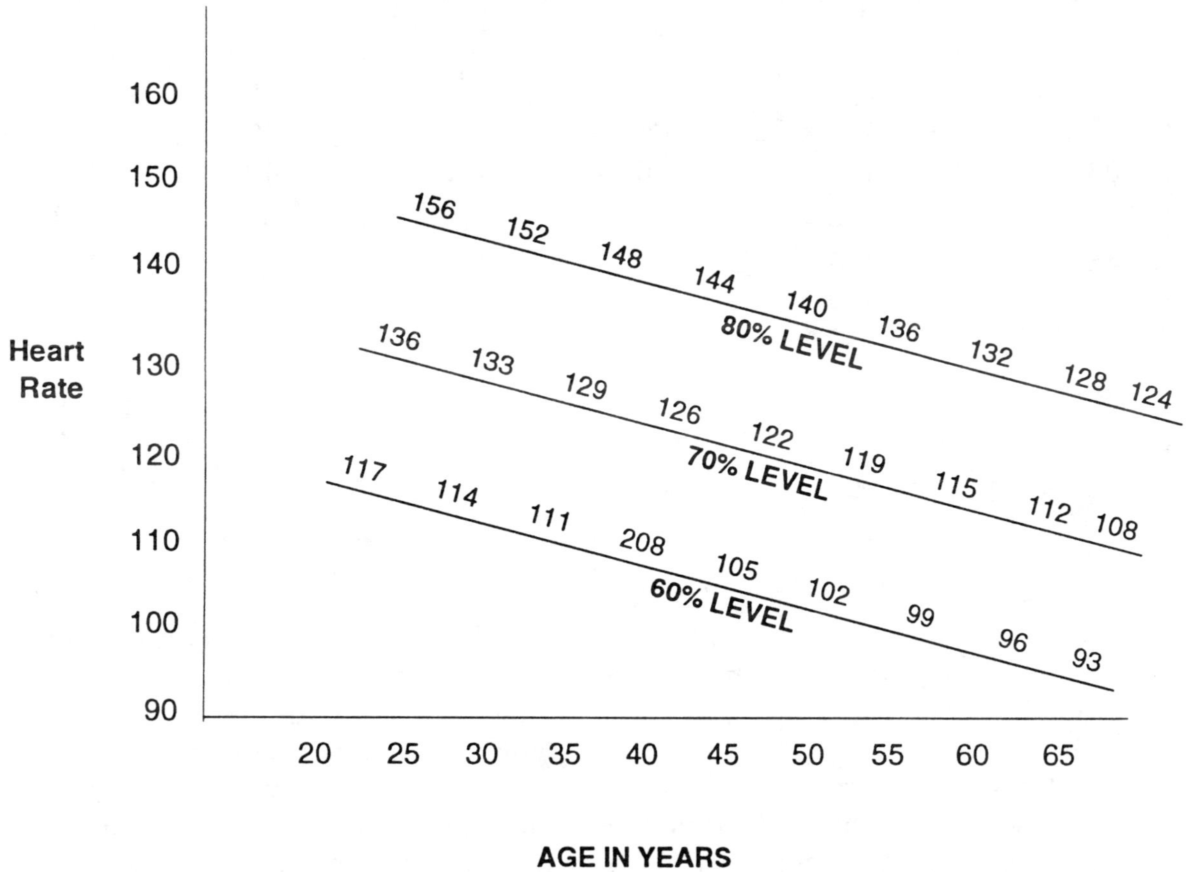

HEART RATES FOR AEROBIC TRAINING PROGRAM

TARGET HEART RATES FOR VARIOUS AGES AND INTENSITIES

Your target heart rate is calculated by subtracting your age from 220, and multiplying the result by .60 (or some higher number, depending on your fitness level and/or state of progress). For your convenience, various age groups are calculated for you below.

Age	.60	.65	.70	75	.80
20	120	130	140	150	160
25	117	127	137	147	157
30	114	124	134	144	154
35	111	120	130	140	150
40	108	117	126	135	144
45	105	114	122	131	140
50	102	110	119	128	136
55	99	108	116	124	132
60	96	104	112	120	128
65	93	101	109	117	125
70	90	98	106	114	122

If your exercise requires a **lot** of effort to get your heart rate into your target zone, and if your exercise makes you **very** tired and uncomfortable, lower your target heart rate. If you are one of the few individuals who must make this reduction, feel no guilt! Remember that your exercise program must be fun and enjoyable. If you discover that your heart rate consistently gets too high during exercise, slow down! As you progress through the program, you will eventually be able to increase your workload. It is much safer to be certain that your progression is reasonable and within your physical capabilities. The ideal aerobic workout should follow the guidelines included in the chart on the following page.

A good exercise program is one that accelerates the heart for a minimum of 20 minutes at the target heart rate for that individual. The target heart rate for someone who is extremely fit, the appropriate target heart rate would be determined by (220-persons age x .80). The example in the chart above is for a person approximately 44 years of age, with no serious health problems, and in a good state of fitness.

The guidelines for an aerobic workout are valid only for those activities we classify as aerobic. The strength program and the flexibility program should be developed in accordance with principles other than heart rates.

AEROBIC EXERCISE TRAINING PROGRAM

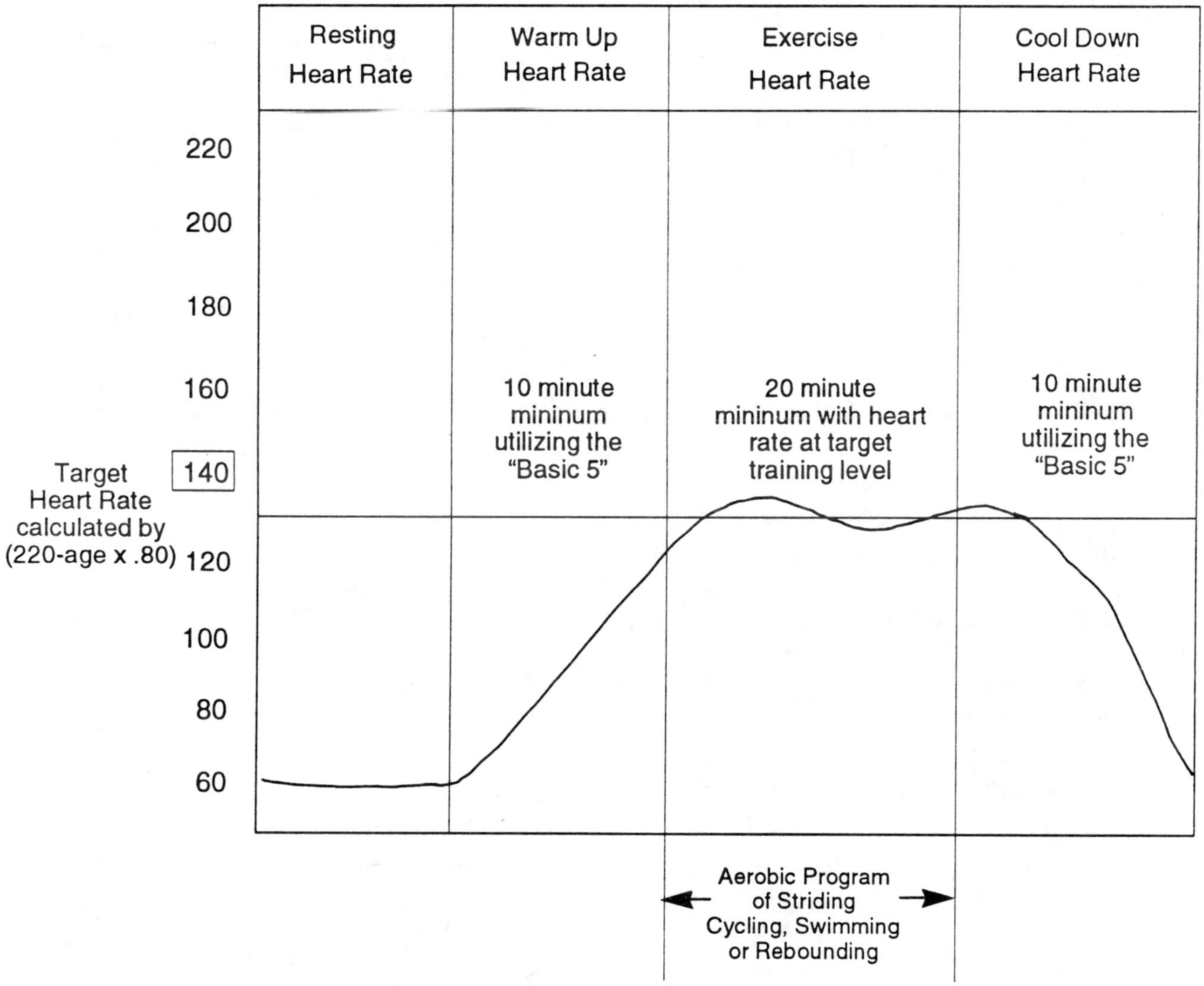

ESTIMATING FITNESS LEVELS BASED ON CURRENT ACTIVITY

		Score
I. How Hard (Intensity)	Sustained heavy breathing and perspiration (Jogging)	5
	Intermittent heavy breathing and perspiration—(Tennis)	4
	Moderate activity—(Recreational sports and easy cycling)	3
	Easy activities—(Volleyball, Softball)	2
	Very easy activities—(Fishing)	1
II. How Long (Duration)	Over 30 minutes	4
	20-30 minutes	3
	10-20 minutes	2
	Under 10 minutes	1
III. How Often (Frequency)	5 times per week or more	5
	3 or 4 times per week	4
	1 or 2 times per week	3
	Few times each month	2
	Less than once a month	1

Your Score = How Hard ________ X How Long ________ X How Often ________

Your category = 80 — Excellent! Keep doing what you're doing and use this manual for information

60-80—High Fitness Level
40-60—Good Fitness Level
Below 40—Average Fitness Level

RESTING HEART RATE CHART

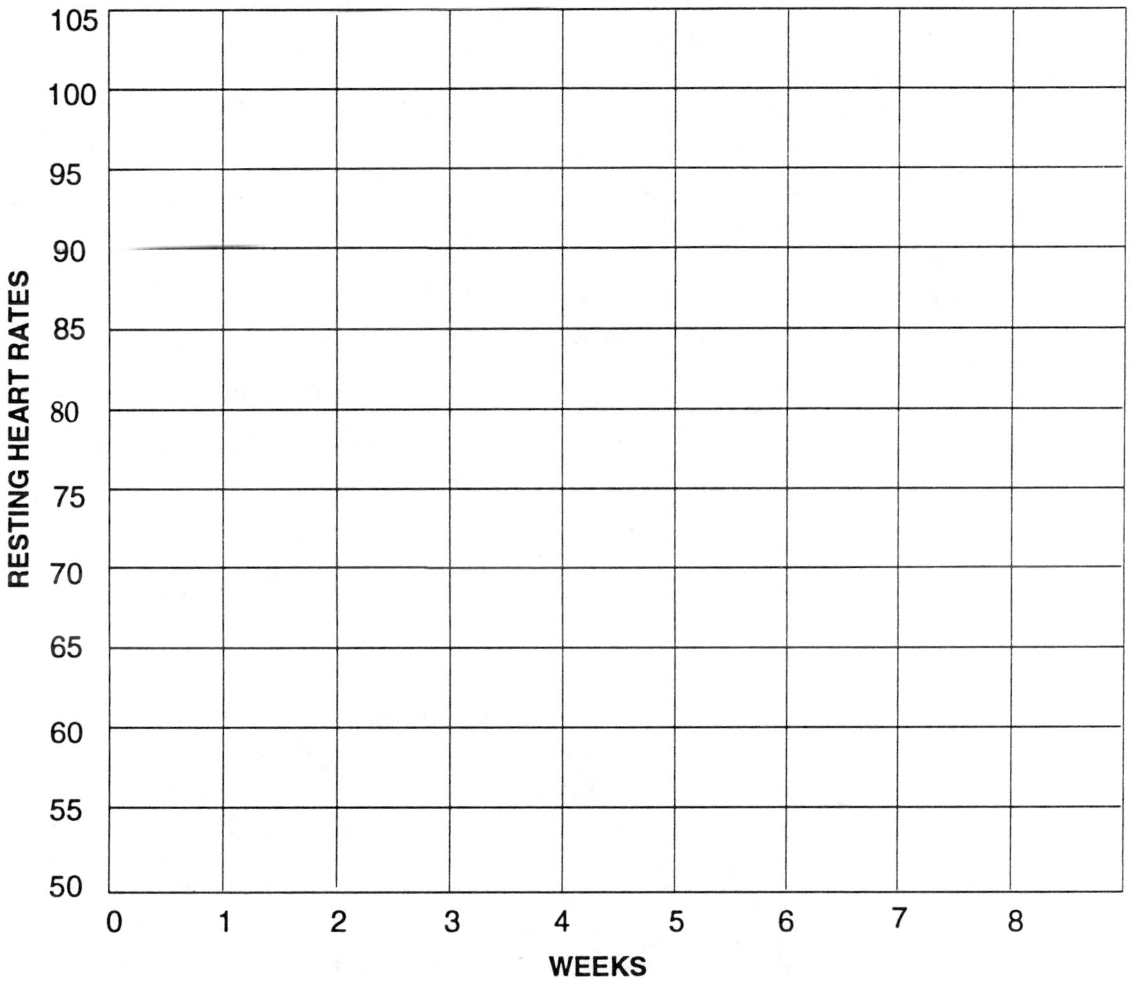

AVERAGE RESTING HEART RATE FOR AN EIGHT WEEK AEROBIC FITNESS PROGRAM

It is not unusual for someone to lower their Resting Heart Rate by as much as 8 beats per minute through involvement in an Eight Week Aerobic Fitness Program. The Resting Heart Rate is one of the best indicators of the health condition of the heart, lungs, and blood vessels. Generally, the lower the Resting Heart Rate, the stronger and healthier the heart. Well trained, conditioned athletes, frequently have Resting Heart Rates in the 40's and 50's. Untrained, poorly conditioned people usually have Resting Heart Rates in the 80's and 90's.

You will average your Resting Heart Rate for each of the next eight weeks and plot this average accordingly on the Average Resting Heart Rate Chart. It will be encouraging and motivating for you to see your Resting Heart Rate decrease as the pumping efficiency of your heart improves from week to week.

Nutritionists generally agree that the average American's diet is poor in spite of the availability of good wholesome food. Most of us are so poorly educated about nutrition that we do not realize the damage we may be doing to our bodies if we eat too much saturated fat, too much sugar, and too many calories. The alarming fact is that these violations of good nutritional habits are contributing to an increased incidence of obesity, heart disease, diabetes, and diseases of the digestive system.

The Senate Select Committee on Nutrition and Human Needs published a report that contains seven important recommendations for improving the nutritional status of the American public. These recommendations were:

1. Eat a variety of foods.
2. Choose a diet low in fat, saturated fat, and cholesterol.
3. Choose a diet with plenty of vegetables, fruits, and grain products.
4. Maintain a healthy weight.
5. Use salt or sodium only in moderation.
6. Use sugars only in moderation.
7. If you drink alcoholic beverages, do so in moderation.

Good Nutrition For Better Fitness

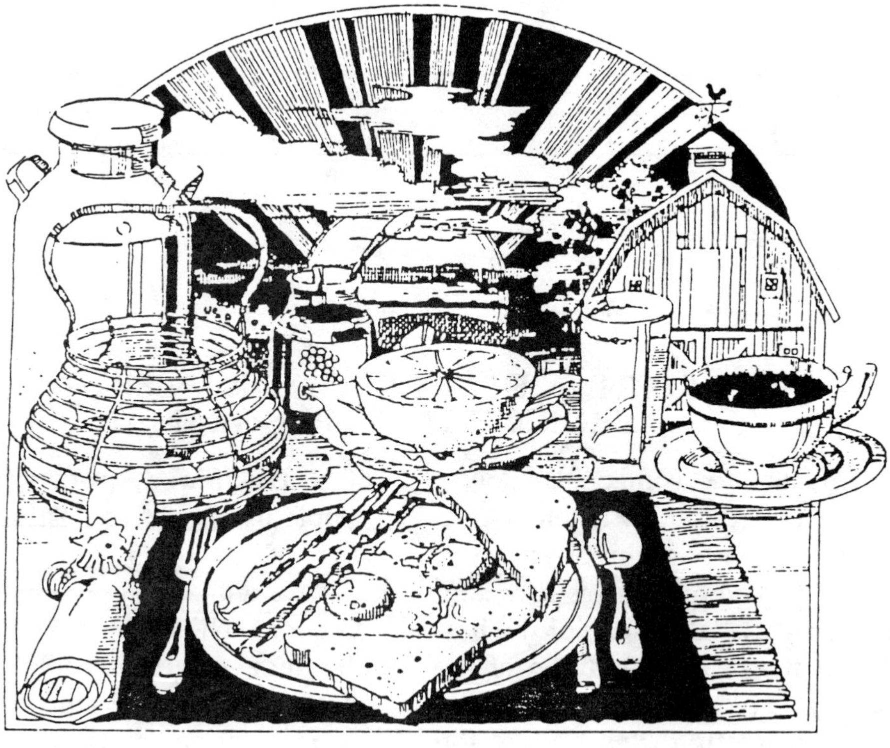

If these adjustments could be implemented, the incidence of disease frequently associated with dietary imbalance would be certain to decrease within the general population. A comparison of the average American's diet and the recommended diet suggested in the "Dietary Goals for the United States" report is as follows:

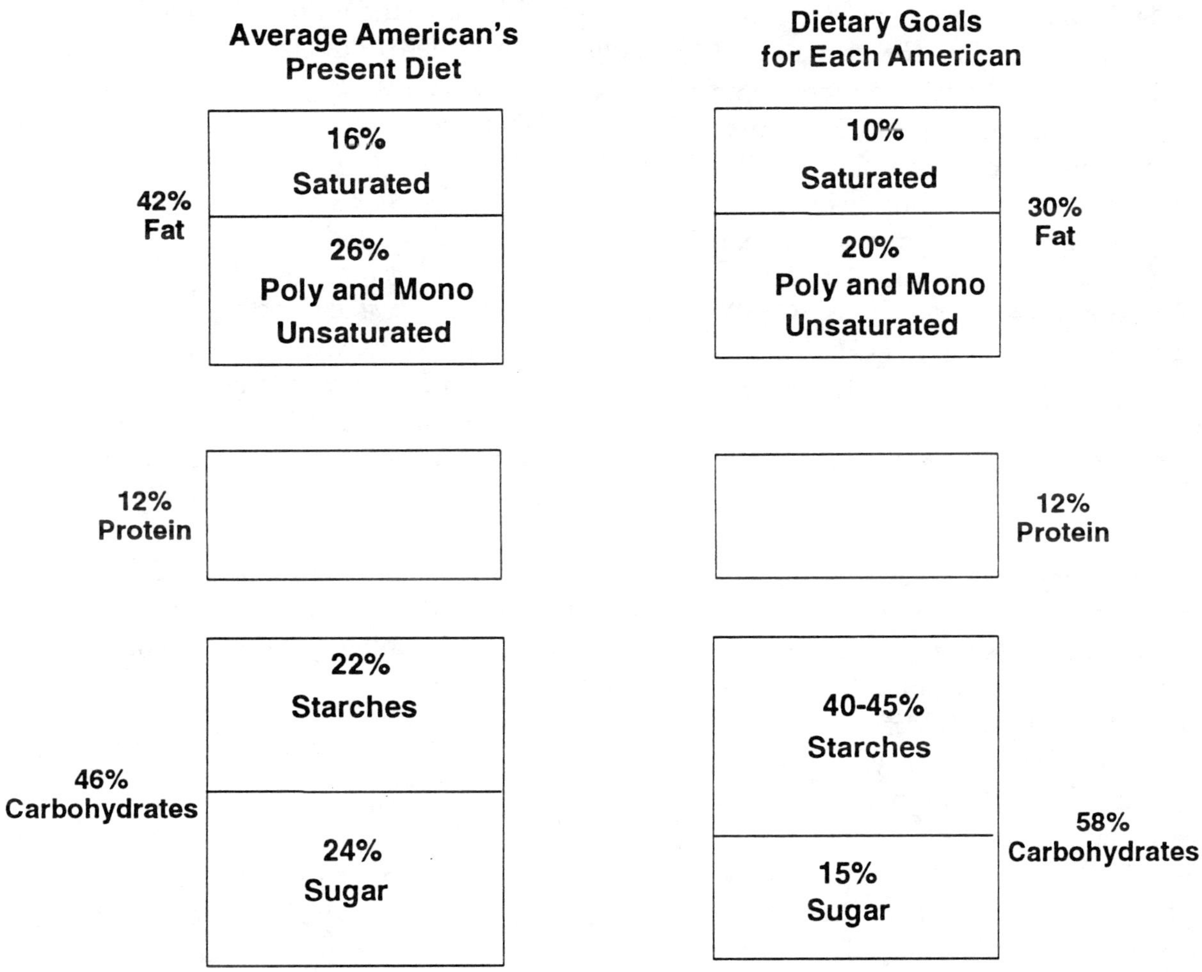

Good nutrition is essential for good health. Daily regular exercise represents only about half of the behaviors fundamental for a healthy body. Good eating habits must also be a primary consideration. To be healthy, your body needs more than forty nutrients which are supplied by six food components: water, carbohydrates, fats, proteins, vitamins, and minerals.

The Six Nutrients

Proteins

Protein is the basic component of the cells of your body necessary for growth and maintenance. Your body produces some amino acids, the building blocks of protein, while others must be supplied by protein enriched foods. Good sources of protein are eggs, dairy products, meat, fish, poultry, beans and nuts. Due to the high fat and cholesterol content of milk, dairy products, nuts and eggs, it is advisable to supply your body with essential amino acids by eating lean meats, fish, poultry, and beans. These foods are very high in protein but contain low levels of fat and cholesterol.

Muscles are composed of protein; therefore, proponents of the "protein myth" believe protein supplements and diets rich in lean red meat builds stronger muscles. Unlike carbohydrates and fats, protein cannot be stored in your body. If you take in more protein then your body requires, you will force your liver and kidneys to be overworked.

Exercise does not increase the body's requirement for protein. A well balanced diet will provide you with all the necessary protein for optimal health and physical performance. Proteins do not provide quick energy nor do they improve your physical stamina.

A meal very rich in protein can cause you to feel tired and fatigued. Excess amounts of protein require energy in order to be adequately diverted into amino acids within the digestive system. It is sensible to maintain a daily dietary intake of 4-8 ounces of good proteins each day.

If you are a vegetarian and desire to receive all of your amino acids each day, you should utilize the following combinations of vegetables products:

**beans and sesame*
**beans and corn*
**beans and rice*
**rice and sesame*
**rice, soybean, and wheat*
**beans and wheat*
**peanuts, wheat, and milk*
**peanuts, soybeans, and sesame*
**greens and converted rice*
**peanuts and sunflower seeds*

Legumes (beans and peas) are low in two essential amino acids that are abundant in grains, and grains are low in two amino acids that are plentiful in legumes. If you will use these guidelines, you will be assured of obtaining all of the essential amino acids.

Fats

Fats are essential in proper quantities for good health. Fats are a primary source of energy at rest. They provide energy during the later stages of an aerobic activity after the muscles have depleted their glycogen supply. Aside from being a good source of energy, fats provide padding around vital organs, and act as an insulation in regulating body temperature. An active person stores fat in the muscles; however, sedentary people store fat in a layer under the skin. A skin fold test can measure the amount of fat under your skin and give you an indication of how much excess fat you are carrying around.

Excess body fat can be harmful and sometimes life threatening. Fat causes obesity, heart failure, diabetes, hypertension and kidney failure. Diets rich in fats usually cause high levels of cholesterol in the blood. Cholesterol is manufactured naturally by the body and is essential for the production of many hormones. Diets rich in fats will overload your cholesterol needs and contribute to the formation of plaque in the arteries. Clogged arteries are a major factor in the development of arteriosclerosis, heart attack and strokes.

Fats are classified as saturated, polyunsaturated, and monounsaturated. Saturated fats are primarily found in animal meats, whole milk, cream, butter, cheese, eggs and lard. Other saturated fats are derived from coconut oil, chocolate, margarine, olives, avocados and nuts. Polyunsaturated fats are usually manufactured from plants and are thought to lower the level of cholesterol in the blood. These polyunsaturated fats are liquid oils found in corn, cottonseed, soybeans, safflower, and sunflower seeds. Monounsaturated fats include peanut oil and olive oil and are now believed to provide health benefits.

A pre- exercise meal, rich in fats, will make you feel sluggish and slow. For optimal health, it is advisable to limit your intake of saturated fats. Charts provided on the following pages will help you plan a good fat modified diet which will help lower your cholesterol level.

HOW TO IMPLEMENT A FAT MODIFIED DIET

KEEPING THE SATURATED FATS DOWN

By using skim milk and by avoiding cream, ice cream, butter, cheese, and other dairy products made from cream or whole milk, you will have already eliminated a large amount of cholesterol and saturated fat from your diet.

You can eliminate still more saturated fat through careful selection and preparation of meat. Here are some tips to help you choose and cook meat to give a minimum of standard fat.

SELECTING MEATS

The lean cuts of beef are the ones to look for—those with more muscle than fat, such as round, rump, and tenderloin. Avoid cuts such as rib roast and steaks in which the fat is distributed throughout the and cannot be removed.

Once you have selected your meat, have the butcher trim away all visible fat. When you get home, cut off and discard any he may have missed.

Have hamburger ground to order from lean round or lean chuck. Do not buy it already ground unless it is in packages especially marked **lean** ground meat. This is sold by some markets at a slightly higher price.

Veal cutlets and chops, and veal steaks, are good choices, because they are so lean. So are veal roasts.

Do not buy canned or frozen cooked meat dishes. You have no way of knowing how much fat, or what kind of fat, they contain.

Remember that fish, chicken, turkey, and cornish hens are good selections because they contain less fat than most meats.

WATER

Most of us do not consider water essential for good health. You might be able to safely omit some of the other nutrients for a few days, but without water you could not survive.

Water composes 70 percent of our bodies. The average person will lose two to three quarts daily through perspiration, vapor from the lungs, urine and feces. Some fluid requirements are provided by the foods we eat; however, even if you do not exercise daily, your body requires **a minimum of six glasses of fluids each day.**

When you exercise, even at a low level of intensity, your body loses fluids. It is good advice to drink plenty of fluids prior to any exercise workout. After you have begun exercising, your body will not be able to absorb fluids at the same rate at which they are being expended. If your body is not properly stocked with fluids during physical exertion you may experience nausea, cramping, or general weakness. It is always good practice to start your exercise program with an extra supply of fluids in your system. This is especially important during hot weather when your body will be perspiring more and losing fluids more readily.

Carbohydrates

Carbohydrates are essential for the functioning of the body. They serve as a source of energy and are necessary for the burning of fats. Carbohydrates provide the body with the best source of energy during physical activity. Food sources for carbohydrates are cereals, bread, rice, pasta, potatoes, fruits and fruit juices. These food sources of carbohydrates are slowly converted into glucose by the body and provide you with a long term energy source.

Simple carbohydrates like table sugar and honey contain glucose in a form that is so quickly absorbed it goes into the bloodstream almost immediately. These pure carbohydrates provide a quick energy source because they trigger the release er level of insulin in the blood. Within a short time your blood sugar level drops andyou may become weak or dizzy. This condition is called rebound hypoglycemia.

Other problems associated with too much sugar in the diet are dental cavities, obesity, irritability, and increased triglyceride levels. A high level of triglycerides in the blood, is recognized as a contributing factor in heart disease.

Many people believe they are avoiding the hazards of "white refined sugar" by using honey, brown sugar or molasses. These are merely substitutes for sugar and initiate the same responses in our bodies as refined sugar.

Vitamins

Vitamins are compounds which are needed in small amounts by your body for normal growth and development. Since our bodies do not manufacture vitamins, they must be obtained through food or supplements. The two basic groups of vitamins are fat soluble and water soluble. Fat soluble vitamins include vitamins A, D, E, and K. These vitamins are in rich supply in liver, eggs, butter, and meat. Water soluble vitamins include vitamin C and the B complex. These vitamins are supplied by fruits, vegetables, grains, beans, and lean meats. In addition, milk contains a generous supply of both water soluble and fat soluble vitamins.

Vitamins are found in almost any food you eat with the exception of sugar. If you diet and take vitamins supplements to provide daily needs, you should be advised that vitamins must be activated by certain nutrients. If your diet is deficient in the required nutrients, the vitamin supplement may be useless.

Ordinarily, vitamin supplements for someone who is healthy, with no apparent signs of disease, is probably unnecessary provided the individual eats two or three balanced meals each day. Specific examples of situations where vitamin supplementation may be necessary include: pregnant or lactating women, individuals under severe stress, people who have recognized deficiencies, people who do not eat balanced meals, people who eat foods that have lost their nutritional value through storage or poor preparation, or individuals who have absorption or utilization problems.

Also, some people have genetic characteristics that alter that individual's vitamin needs and those people may require supplementation. Of course, all the factors that could create the need for vitamin supplementation have not been clearly identified. For this reason, some people take vitamin and mineral supplements as a purely precautionary measure.

It is important for you to know what vitamins "will" and "will not" do. Even though it is true that vitamins are essential for good health, vitamins can be harmful if taken in excessive amounts or in the wrong proportions. Massive doses of vitamins will not necessarily make you "super healthy"; however, when deficiencies exist, vitamins can help solve many health problems.

While vitamin supplementation is necessary for some individuals, it should remain the responsibility of a doctor skilled at diagnosing nutritional deficiency and prescribing appropriate supplementation. Review the following charts in an effort to more fully understand the relationship of vitamins to health and fitness.

RECOMMENDED DIETARY ALLOWANCES

(RDA), 1989

	Males			Females		
Age (yrs.)	15-18	19-24	25-50	15-18	19-24	25-50
Protein (g)	59	58	63	44	46	50
Vitamin A (RE)	1000	1000	1000	800	800	800
Vitamin D (ug)	10	10	5	10	10	5
Vitamin E (mg)	10	10	10	8	8	8
Vitamin K (ug)	65	70	80	55	60	65
Vitamin C (mg)	60	60	60	60	60	60
Thiamin (mg)	1.5	1.5	1.5	1.1	1.1	1.1
Riboflavin (mg)	1.8	1.7	1.7	1.3	1.3	1.3
Niacin (mg equiv.)	20	19	19	15	15	15
Vitamin B6 (mg)	2.0	2.0	2.0	1.5	1.5	1.5
Folacin (ug)	200	200	200	180	180	180
Vitamin B12 (ug)	2.0	2.0	2.0	2.0	2.0	2.0
Calcium (mg)	1200	1200	800	1200	1200	800
Phosphorous (mg)	1200	1200	800	1200	1200	800
Magnesium (mg)	400	350	350	300	280	280
Iron (mg)	12	10	10	15	15	15
Zinc (mg)	15	15	15	12	12	12
Iodine (ug)	150	150	150	150	150	150
Selenium (ug)	50	70	70	50	55	55

Source: Dept. of Health and Human Services, Food and Drug Administration, Washington, D.C.

1.

Vitamin	Sources	Advantages	Symptoms of Deficiencies
A	Fish Yellow-green vegetables Green leafy vegetables Spinach Apricots Carrots Dairy Products Egg Yolks	Promotes healthy eyes Promotes healthy skin Promotes healthy hair Protects membranes and lungs from infections Aids absorbtion of proteins Aids urinary tract	Menstrual problems Dry and cracked skin Eye inflammation (sites, glare blindness, night blindness, dryness) Eruptions around hair follicles Lack of appetite Respiratory infections Headaches
People Most Prone to Deficiencies: Cigarette smokers, marijuana smokers, drug users, alcoholics, newborn babies, nursing mothers, individuals using eyes excessively, fat defficient diets.			

2.

Vitamin	Sources	Advantages	Symptoms of Deficiencies
B[1]	Beef Pork Milk Cereal Grains, cereals and breads Nuts	Promotes emotional stability Aids digestion Helps prevent fatigue Promotes growth (in children) Helps strengthen heart muscle Reduces hardening of the arteries	Mucous membrane irritations Diarrhea Itrritability Depression Emotional instability Loss of alertness
People Most Prone to Deficiencies: Alcoholics, cigarette smokers, arthritic individuals, overstressers, heavy laborers, pregnant women, irregular eaters.			

3.

Vitamins	Sources	Advantages	Symptoms of Deficiencies
B[2] (Riboflavin)	Fish Eggs Liver Red Meat Green vegetables Whole grain breads and cereal	Aids breakdown of fats and proteins Relieves depression Increases energy	Tongue inflammation (glossitis) Bloodshot eyes Eyes over-sensitive to light Itchy, dry skin Anemia
People Most Prone to Deficiencies: Depressed individuals, elderly people, women using oral contraceptives, irregular eaters, overstressed and tense individuals.			

4.

Vitamins	Sources	Advantages	Symptoms of Deficiencies
B[3] (Niacin)	Fish Lean meats Milk Green leafy vegetables Peanuts Eggs	Aids breakdown and utilization of proteins and fats Reduces cholesterol Improves circulaton Improves health of skin Helps balance sex hormones Maintains healthy nerves	Diarrhea Insomnia Irritability Dermatitis Depression Fatigue Headaches Emotional moodiness Lack of concentration Halitosis
People Most Prone to Deficiencies: Hypoglycemics, antibiotic users, overusers of sugar and starches, individuals with high cholesterol levels, over stressed individuals.			

5.

Vitamins	Sources	Advantages	Symptoms of Deficiencies
B^5 (Pantothenic acid)	Molasses Eggs Cabbage Peas Liver Green leafy vegetables	Aids metabolism of fats and proteins Helps prevent arthritis Improves skin (helps prevent wrinkles) Stimulates adrenal glands Balances blood sugar Helps prevent fatigue Aids body's thermo insulation Helps prevent premature aging Aids stress management	Stomach disturbances Anxiety Mental confusion Fatigue Skin/hair disorders Low blood sugar Hypoglycemia Upper respiratory infections

People Most Prone to Deficiencies: Heavy sugar users, antibiotic users, hypoglycemics, over stressed individuals, cold climate laborers, arthritics.

6.

Vitamins	Sources	Advantages	Symptoms of Deficiencies
B^6 (Pyridoxine)	Peas Lean Meats Whole grain Cereals Eggs Beans	Aids in breakdown of fats Helps control cholesterol levels Aids metabolism Helps prevent water retention in tissues	Glossitis Dermatitis Increased susceptibility to infection Depression Irritability Emotional instability Swelling of stomach, hands, feet Hair loss

People Most Prone to Defeciencies: Alcoholics, over stressed individuals, dieting or fasting individuals, pregnant women, nursing mothers, older people, people with high protein diets.

7. Vitamins	Sources	Advantages	Symptoms of Defficiencies
B^{12} (Cyanocobalim)	Oysters Saltwater Fish Liver Beef Eggs Milk	Helps prevent anemia Promotes growth in children Helps utilization of protein and fats	Moodiness Anemia Stunted growth Fatigue Sore, weak muscles Mental slowness Spinal cord degeneration
People Most Prone to Deficiencies: Women with irregular menstruation, excessive laxative users, older people, nonmeat eaters (vegetarians)			

8. Vitamins	Sources	Advantages	Symptoms of Defficiencies
Folic Acid	Mushrooms Milk Meat Liver Brewer's yeast Green leafy vegetables Wheat bran	Helps form red blood cells Improves circulation Promotes formation of proteins Aids digestion of proteins Aids absorption of A, D, E, K vitamins	Anemia Graying Hair Premature birth Gastrointestinal disturbances Lack of appetite
People Most Prone to Deficiencies: Over stressed individuals, diabetics, alcoholics, sulfa drug users, pregnant women, older people, women with excessive menstrual flow.			

9. Vitamins	Sources	Advantages	Symptoms of Deficiencies
C	Citrus Fruits Tomatoes Potatoes Green peppers Cantaloupe Strawberries Green leafy vegetables	Helps prevent colds Helps reduce allergies Aids healing of wounds and burns Strengthens blood vessels Aids metobalism of calcium and amino acids Aids absorption of iron Helps reduce fatigue and stress Aids stamina Helps strengthen bones and teeth	Anemia Weakness Nose bleeds Spongy gums Frequent colds Soreness of muscles and joints Shortness of breath Slow healer Skin disordeers (acne, psoriasis)

People Most Prone to Deficiencies: Alcoholics, cigarette smokers, antibiotic users, older people, lacking fresh fruit and vegetables in diet, heroine users, individuals with excessive eye strain.

10. Vitamins	Sources	Advantages	Symptoms of Deficiencies
D	Salmon Fortified milk Egg yolks Liver Enriched cereals Sunshine Sardines	Helps promote growth Strengthens bones and teeth Aids normal growth Aids absorption of calcium and phosporus Improves nervous system	Eye strain Hypoparathyroidism Flabbiness Dental cavities Stomach ulcers Excessive colds and flu Rickets

People Most Prone to Deficiencies: Pregnant women, individuals who read excessively, individuals with heart disease.

11. Vitamins	Sources	Advantages	Symptoms of Deficiencies
E	Whole-grain cereals Vegetable oils Wheat germ Raw peanuts Cottonseed oil	Helps regulate menstrual rhythm Helps prevent miscarriage Helps prevent blood clotting Aids metabolism of calcium and protein Promotes healthy skin Helps strengthen capillary walls Helps prevent scarring Helps lower cholesterol and fatty acids Improves circulation	Anemia in premature babies Elevated cholesterol Headaches

People Most Prone to Deficiencies: User of unsaturated oils, drinkers of highly chlorinated water, over stressed individuals, premature babies, pregnant women, nursing mothers, infants, older people.

12. Vitamins	Sources	Advantages	Symptoms of Deficiencies
K	Milk Yogurt Fruit Cauliflower Alfalfa Kelp	Aids normal liver functions Natural painkiller Helps enhance vitality Promotes longevity Aids conversion of glucose into glycogen	Excessive bleeding

People Most Prone to Deficiencies: Overusers of aspirins, older persons, antibiotic users, individuals who eat excessive amounts of frozen foods, individuals with poor bile secretions.

13. Vitamins	Sources	Advantages	Symptoms of Deficiencies
P (Bioflavenoids)	Citrus fruit Apricots Cherries Strawberries Cantaloupe Tomatoes Blackberries Grapes Cabbage Cauliflower Leafy vegetables	Aids absorption of vitamin C Helps strengthen capillaries Helps protect against x-rays Helps prevent colds and flu Lowers blood pressure Helps prevent hardening of arteries	Tendency to bleed easily (nosebleeds) (gum bleeding) Bruising easily Soreness of joints and muscles Fatigue
People Most Prone to Deficiencies: Overweight individuals, diabetics, x-ray technicians, individuals with high blood pressure, over stressed individuals, individuals with respiratory infections.			

MINERALS

Minerals are essential for building bones, teeth, blood, nerve cells, and muscles. They also help your body regulate water and acid levels.

Minerals are found in the soil and are absorbed from the soil by plants. When we eat plants the minerals are incorporated into our bodies. Minerals must be supplied daily because they are not stored in our bodies.

Calcium, iodine, potassium, and magnesium are the four basic minerals our bodies require in large amounts. There are fourteen other minerals that are needed in trace amounts. Science has not developed a pill that contains all eighteen minerals in the proper proportions. The best way to satisfy your body's need for minerals is through a well balanced diet with a variety of fruits, nuts, vegetables, cereals, dairy and poultry products. These foods should provide your basic mineral needs, without the expense of mineral supplements.

1.

Minerals	Sources	Advantages	Symptoms of Deficiencies
Calcium	Milk Dairy Products Leafy green vegetables (spinach, broccoli, mustard greens, etc.)	Helps promote healthy bones and teeth Promotes healthy skin Helps decrease insomnia Aids absorption of iron Assist blood clotting Helps relieve pain Helps relieve cramps Assists muscle contraction	Muscle cramps Insomnia Skin erruptions Elevated heart rate Pains in joints Calcium deposits in joints and tissues
People Most Prone to Deficiencies: Over stressed individuals, arthritics, over users of laxatives, alcoholics, over users of vitamins A, C, D, sedentary indiviuals, over eaters of chocolate, women suffering from dysmenorrhea.			

2.

Minerals	Sources	Advantages	Symptoms of Deficiencies
Copper	Almonds Sea foods Liver Whole grain cereals; breads Green leafy vegetables	Helps form hemoglobin and red blood cells Aids absorption of iron Facilitates healing aids metabolism of proteins Forms hair pigments	Fatigue Anemia White spotting on fingernails Difficulty breathing Skin eruptions
People Most Prone to Deficiencies: Anemics, excessive bleeders			

3.

Minerals	Sources	Advantages	Symptoms of Deficiencies
Iodine	Sea food Iodized salt Kelp Mushrooms	Promotes a healthy thyroid gland Helps the body burn fats Promotes healthy hair, fingernails, skin and teeth Facilitates growth	Nervousness Slow metabolism Goiter formation Sluggishness Irritability Hardening of the arteries Dry hair and scalp
People Most Prone to Deficiencies: Excessive perspirers, people living where soil is depleted, users of uniodized salt.			

4.

Mineral	Sources	Advantages	Symptoms of Deficiencies
Iron	Lean meat Green leafy vegetables Liver Oysters	Aids absorption of protein and copper Helps form hemoglobin	Anemia Fatigue Difficulty breathing Paleness of skin Brittle fingernails Constipation
People Most Prone to Deficiencies: Pregnant women, women during menstruation, individuals experiencing rapid growth, peptic ulcers sufferers, individuals losing large amounts of blood, individuals with a low vitamin C diet.			

5.

Mineral	Sources	Advantages	Symptoms of Deficiencies
Magnesium	Apples Nuts Wheat germ Green vegetables Soybeans Figs	Helps prevent tooth decay Facilitates formation of tooth enamel Helps regulate body temperature Promotes growth of bones Promotes the absorption of other vitamins & minerals Helps reduce cholesterol Helps lessen depression Helps prevent calcium deposits	Depression Mental disorientation Muscle twitches Low body temperature

People Most Prone to Deficiencies: Diabetics, excessive sugar users, people with poor eating habits, alcoholics, pregnant women, nursing mothers, diuretic users, people on high protein diets.

6.

Mineral	Sources	Advantages	Symptoms of Deficiencies
Phosphorus	Eggs Nuts Meat Fish Poultry Whole grain cereal & bread	Facilitates growth of teeth and bones Promotes healing of bones Aids absorption of B-complex vitamins Promotes mental & physical efficiency Helps break down fats	Loss of appetite Fatigue

People Most Prone to Deficiencies: Pregnant women, growing children, over stressed individuals, cancer victims, arthritics, over users of laxatives.

7.

Mineral	Sources	Advantages	Symptoms of Deficiencies
Potassium	Bananas Oranges Potatoe skins Meats Green leafy vegetables Whole grain cereals & breads Sunflower seeds	Promotes healthy skin Regulates body's water balance Converts glucose into glucose Helps regulate heartbeat Facilitates growth	Irregular heartbeat Skin eruptions Insomnia Fatigue Poor reflexes Constipation Headaches Muscular weakness
People Most Prone to Deficiencies: Excessive salt users, excessive coffee drinkers, alcoholics, over stressed individuals, older people, people with high blood pressure, over users of laxatives, diuretic users, excessive perspirers, hypoglycemics, migraine headache sufferers, cortisone users, diarrhea sufferers.			

8.

Mineral	Sources	Advantages	Symptoms of Deficiencies
Zinc	Bran Meats Fish Poultry Cereal Spinach Eggs	Promotes healthy hair Helps decrease cholesterol Aids manufacturing of insulin Facilitates growth Helps promote healing Aids absorption of B-complex Helps function of prostrate gland Helps prevent sterility	Mental dullness Loss of appetite Fatigue Unhealthy skin Slower healer Hypogonadism Dull hair
People Most Prone to Deficiencies: Alcoholics, oral contraceptive users, pregnant women, cancer victims, diabetics, men with prostrate problems, over emotional individuals.			

WEIGHT LOSS PROFILE

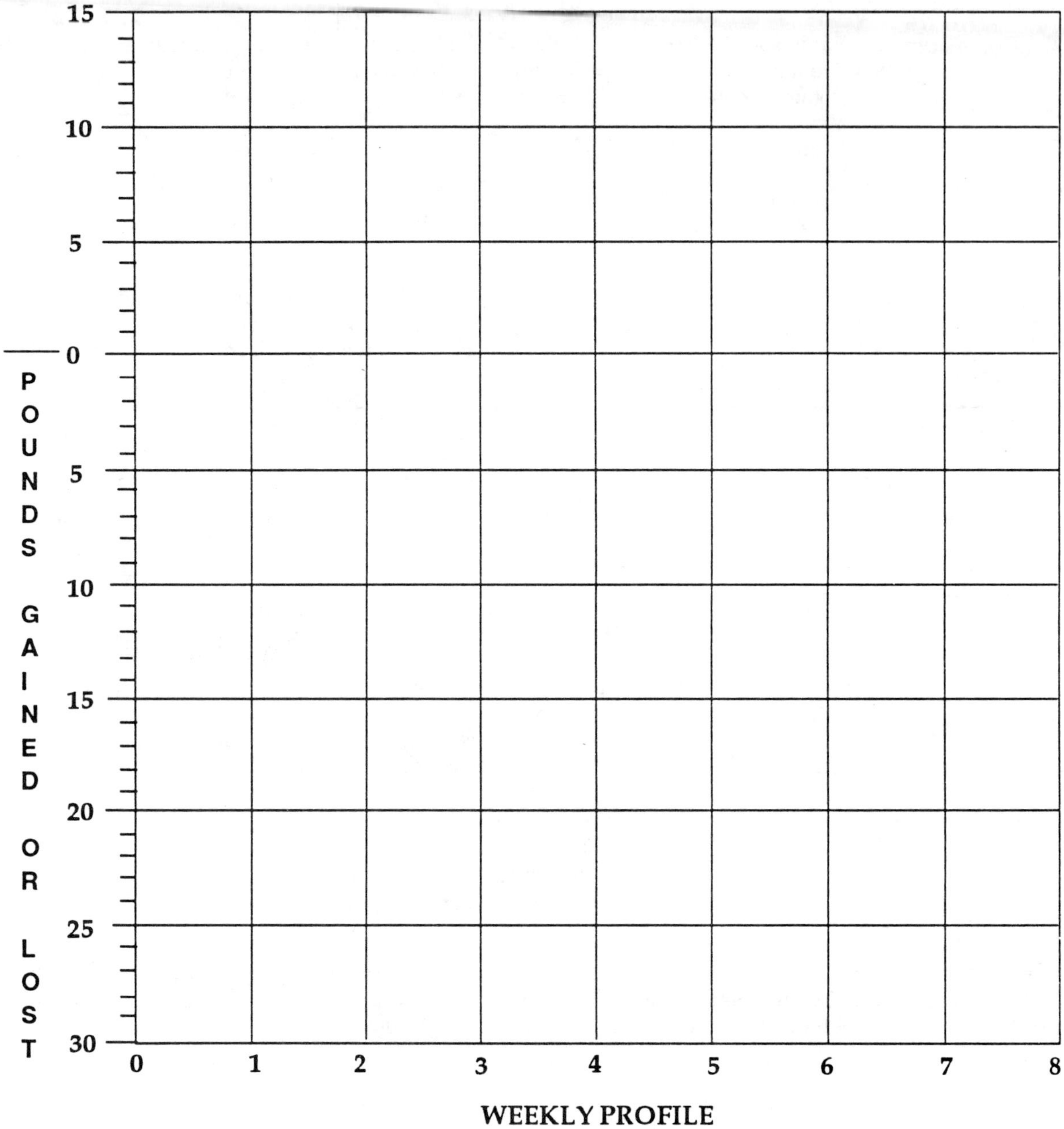

1. Write your current weight beside the "0" point and plot the "0" point to represent your present weight as you begin this program.
2. Each **week** weigh yourself and plot your weight loss for the appropriate day.
3. Connect the points with a line to see your profile as you lose weight through this program.

Caloric Values of Common Foods

Food	Amount	Grams of Fat	Calories
Abalone	4 oz.	.8	91
Anchovies	5 fillets	1.9	35
Apples	1 medium	.5	80
Apple Butter	1 tbsp.	.2	37
Applesauce			
unsweetened	1/2 cup	.1	50
sweetened	1/2 cup	.2	115
Apples, dried unsweetened	1/2 cup	.2	115
Apple juice,	8 oz. glass	.1	117
Apricots			
canned in heavy syrup	1/2 cup	.1	110
dried, cooked (unsweetened)	1/2 cup	.1	125
dried, uncooked	1/2 cup (20 halves)	.1	195
fresh	3	.4	55
Artichoke hearts (Birds Eye)	3 hearts	.1	22
Asparagus			
canned	6 spears	.8	22
raw	1/2 pound	1.0	33
Avocados	1/2 of a 10 oz. avocado	15.0	195
Bacon	2 med. slices	8.0	85
broiled	2 thin slices	6.2	60
Canadian	1 slice	4.2	58
Bananas	1 medium	.5	85
Bass			
Sea	4 oz.	2.3	106
Striped	4 oz.	3.0	120
White	4 oz.	2.4	112
Beans			
baked (with molasses & pork)	4 oz.	3.0	106
barbequed	4 oz.	2.8	124
green, whole (Birds Eye)	1/2 cup	.2	20
lima, immature, cooked, drained	1/2 cup	.5	93
red kidney, canned (solids & liquid)	1/2 cup	.5	115
Beef			
brisket (lean only)	4 oz.	14.4	253
club steak (lean only)	4 oz.	7.2	278
pot pie with vegetables	1 pie 4-1/4" across	33.0	560
pot roasted (lean only)	3 oz.	3.0	165
pot roasted (lean & fat)	3 oz.	8.0	245
roast (lean & fat)	3 oz.	28.2	375
rump roast (roasted)	4 oz.	22.0	395
T-Bone steak (lean only) broiled	4 oz.	11.9	254
Beef and vegetable stew	1 cup	10.0	210
Beets			
canned (solids & liquid)	1/2 cup	.2	35
green	1/2 cup	.1	15
Biscuits			
home recipe	1 biscuit, 2" diameter	5.0	105
mix	1 biscuit, 2" diameter	3.3	90
Blackberries, fresh	1/2 cup	.3	42
Blueberries, fresh	1/2 cup	.6	45
Bologna or baloney	2 slices (3" dia. x 1/8)	7.0	80
Boysenberries, fresh	1/2 pound	.9	125
Bran, see Cereals			
Braunschweiger	2 oz.	15.2	180
Bread			
Cracked Wheat	1 slice	.9	65
French	1 slice	1.0	58
Italian	1 slice	.2	55

Food	Amount	Grams of Fat	Calories
Pumpernickel	1 slice	.8	74
Raisin	1 slice	1.0	65
Rye	1 slice	.8	60
Vienna	1 slice	1.0	58
Whole Wheat	1 slice	1.0	65
Bread, sweet			
Banana-nut roll	1/2 slice	3.9	71
Date-nut roll	1/2 slice	4.1	75
Broccoli, cut up & drained	1/2 cup	.2	25
Brownie with nuts	1 medium	6.3	90
Brussel sprouts, cooked	1/2 cup	.4	26
Butter or margarine	1 tbsp.	12.0	100
margarine whipped	1 tbsp.	11.0	70
Cabbage			
cooked	1/2 cup	.1	15
raw (shredded)	1/2 cup	.1	7
Cake			
angel food	1 sector, 2-1/2"	.2	135
butter plain (no icing)	3"sq.	12.0	315
butter plain (boiled icing)	1 pc. (1/9 of 9" sq.)	12.0	400
chocolate, chocolate icing	1 sector 2"	9.0	235
fruit, dark	1 pc. (1/9 of 9"sq.)	3.3	55
gingerbread	1 pc. (1/9 of 9" sq.)	7.3	175
pound	1 slice	8.0	
	(1/2"x3-1/2" x3"	9.0	140
sponge	1 slice	4.0	145
Candy			
Almond Joy	1 bar	7.8	247
Almond Cluster	1 bar	12.4	171
Almonds, sugar coated	1 oz.	14.7	128
Buttermint	1 pc.	.1	8
Butterscotch	1 oz.	2.5	111
Caramel, chocolate	1 pc.	1.0	32
Caramel, vanilla	1 pc.	1.0	33
Caravelle	1 bar	6.7	191
Cashew Custer (chocolate covered)	1 pc.	4.4	58
Chocolate milk	1 oz.	9.0	146
Chocolate Almond	1 bar	15.4	250
Chocolate Kisses	1 pc.	1.4	47
Chocolate (semi-sweet)	1 bar	12.4	216
Coconut (chocolate covered)	1 oz.	5.0	122
Life Saver drop	1 pc.	.0	9
Malted Milk Ball	1 pc.	.5	11
Marshmallow	1 medium	.0	26
Mounds	1 bar	14.0	274
Mr. Goodbar	1 bar	19.4	326
Carp, raw, flesh only	4 oz.	6.4	131
Carrots			
cooked, diced	1/2 cup	.1	22
raw	1 medium .1 30		
cooked or canned	1/2 cup	.1	25
Catsup, tomato, bottle	1 tbsp.	.1	18
Cauliflower			
cooked	1/2 cup	.1	15
raw	1/2 pound	.5	61
Caviar, granular	1 oz.	5.8	74
Celery, raw	3 stalks	.3	10
Cereals			
All-Bran	1 cup	1.5	192
Alpha-Bits	1 cup	.7	110
Apple Jacks	1 cup	.1	112
Bran, 100%	1 cup	2.8	150

FOOD	AMOUNT	GRAMS OF FAT	CALORIES
Cereals (*continued*)			
Bran flakes, 40% (Kellog's)	1 cup	.8	139
Bran with raisins	3/4 cup	.7	109
Bran Buds	1 cup	2.1	196
Cap'n Crunch	1 cup	3.5	151
Cheerios	1 cup	.5	100
Cocoa Krispies	1 cup	.6	113
Cocoa Puffs	1 cup	1.0	111
Corn Flakes	1 cup	.5	79
Corn, puffed sweetened	1 oz.	.2	115
Corn, shredded	1 oz.	.2	110
Corn Grits, enriched	3/4 cup	.5	95
Cream of Wheat, cooked	1 cup	.1	110
Crispy Critters	1 cup	.1	110
Froot Loops	1 cup	.5	114
Frosty O's	1 cup	.1	128
Grape-Nuts	1 cup	.4	400
Grape-Nut Flakes	1 cup	.4	150
Kix	1 cup	.4	84
Life	1 cup	2.6	142
Lucky Charms	1 cup	1.1	97
Macaroni, enriched	3/4 cup	.6	115
Macaroni & cheese	1/2 cup	11.0	215
Noodles, enriched	3/4 cup	1.5	150
Oat Flakes	1 cup	1.2	165
Oats, puffed	1 oz.	1.0	115
Oatmeal or rolled oats cooked	1 cup	2.0	130
Oatmeal	3/4 cup	1.7	100
OK's	1 cup	1.0	82
Post Toasties	1 cup	.3	110
Product 19	1 cup	.3	106
Puffed Wheat	1 cup	.2	43
Raisin Bran	1 cup	.8	150
Rice, instant	3/4 cup	.0	135
Rice, shredded	1 oz.	.3	115
Rice, puffed	1 oz.	.1	110
Rice Krispies	1 cup	.2	106
Shredded Wheat, plain	1 biscuit	.3	90
Special K	1 cup	.1	70
Sugar Crisps	1 cup	.3	147
Sugar Frosted Flakes	1 cup	.2	143
Sugar Pops	1 cup	.1	110
Sugar Smacks	1 cup	.7	110
Total	1 cup	.6	108
Trix	1 cup	.4	112
Wheat, rolled, cooked	3/4 cup	.5	135
Wheat Flakes	1 oz.	.3	100
Wheat Germ	1 tbsp.	.5	25
Wheaties	1 cup	.5	108
Cheese			
Blue or Roquefort	1 oz.	9.0	105
Cheddar	1 oz.	9.4	60
Cottage, creamed	1 cup	10.0	260
Cottage, uncreamed	1 cup	2.0	170
Creamed	1 cu. inch	6.0	60
Edam	1 oz.	8.0	105
Food, pasteurized process (American)	1 oz. (slice)	7.0	90
Monterey	1 oz.	8.6	103
Mozzarella	1 oz.	6.1	79
Muenster	1 oz.	8.5	100
Parmesan, grated	1 oz.	1.5	105
processed (American)	1 oz.	9.0	105
processed (American with brick)	1 oz.	8.4	101
Provolone	1 oz.	7.6	99
Romano	1 oz.	7.6	110
spread, pasteurized process	1 oz.	6.0	80
Swiss	1 oz.	8.0	105
Cheese Spread			
American	1 oz.	6.0	81
bacon & horseradish cream cheese	1 oz.	6.0	91
Cheez Whiz	1 oz.	5.7	76
chive cream cheese	1 oz.	6.0	84
Velveeta	1 oz.	6.1	84
Cherries			
maraschino, bottled	2 average	.1	19
red sour, canned (pitted)	1/2 cup	.5	50
Cherry drink (Hi-C)	8 oz. glass	.0	122
Chestnuts, fresh	2 large	.3	29
Chicken			
broiled (no skin)	3 oz.	3.0	115
fried	1/2 breast	12.0	160
	1 thigh	9.5	120
	1 leg	6.0	90
pot pie with vegetables	1 pie, 4-1/4" across	31.0	535
Chili			
with beans	1/2 cup	7.5	170
without beans	1/2 cup	19.0	240
Chocolate, bitter or baking	1 oz.	11.3	143
Chocolate candy, see Candies			
Chocolate drink, mix, powder	3 heaping tsp.	.8	84
Chop suey, with meat, canned	4 oz.	4.0	71
Chow Mein, chicken, without noodles, canned	4 oz.	1.7	43
Clams (meat only)	3 oz.	1.0	65
Cocoa	1 cup	10.8	245
mix, powder	3 heaping tsp.	2.0	73
Coconut, fresh	1 pc. 2"x2" x1/2"	16.0	156
Cod			
broiled with butter	4 oz.	9.2	194
frozen, fillets	2 fillets, 4 oz.	.8	84
Coffee			
prepared, plain	1 cup	.0	2
instant, prepared, plain	1 cup	.0	3
Coleslaw			
with mayonnaise	1/2 cup	7.1	85
with salad dressing	1/2 cup	2.4	60
Collards, cooked	1/2 cup	.5	25
Cookies			
animal crackers	1 pc.	.2	12
chocolate chip	1 pc.	2.2	50
chocolate fudge sandwich	1 pc.	5.0	74
creme sandwich	1 pc.	3.0	50
fig bar	1 pc.	1.0	50
oatmeal	1 pc.	2.6	60
peanut	1 pc.	2.6	33
shortbread	1 pc.	1.7	38
sugar	1 pc.	1.7	35
vanilla wafer	1 pc.	.6	20
Corned beef			
canned	3 oz	14.0	185
mash	3 oz.	11.0	155
Corn			
canned (solids & liquids)	1/2 cup	1.0	85
on the cob, yellow	1 ear, med.	1.0	70
cream style, canned	1/2 cup	.7	105
kernels, canned	1/2 cup	.8	70
Corn chips	1 oz.	8.8	166
Cornbread, mix, prepared	1 pc.	4.0	123
Crab meat	3 oz.	.4	80
fresh, steamed, meat only	4 oz.	1.7	105
canned, drained	1/2 cup	1.0	86
Cracker sandwiches			
packaged cheese peanut butter	1 pc.	1.5	38
Crackers			
butter	1 cracker	1.0	15
cheese	1 cracker	1.0	15
Cheese-Nips	1 cracker	.3	5
Chees Tid-Bits	1 cracker	.4	4
Graham	4 crackers	2.0	
	2-1/2" sq.	1.1	110
Hi-Ho	1 cracker	.3	17
Krispy	1 cracker	.2	12
Melba toast, white	1 cracker	1.0	16

Food	Amount	Grams of Fat	Calories
Crackers (*continued*)			
Ritz	1 cracker	.2	18
Rye	2 wafers	.3	45
Saltines	1 cracker	.4	12
Soda	1 cracker	.4	26
Triscuits	1 cracker	.7	22
White Saltines	4 crackers	1.6	50
Cranberry juice coctail, canned	8 oz. glass	.1	163
Cranberry sauce			
jellied, canned	4 oz.	.2	184
whole, canned	4 oz.	.2	192
Cream			
light	1 tbsp.	3.0	30
half & half	1 tbsp.	2.0	20
heavy whipping	2 tbsp. whipped or 1 tsp. unwhipped	6.0	55
imitation, powdered	1 tsp.	1.0	10
imitation, liquid	1 stp.	2.0	20
sour	1 t bsp.	2.0	25
sour imitation	1 tbsp.	2.0	20
Cucumber, fresh	6 slices, 1/8" thick	.0	5
	1/2 pound	.3	33
Custard, baked	1/2 cup	7.5	150
Dates, dried	1/2 cup	.5	245
Dip onion	1 oz.	4.0	69
Doughnuts			
cake type plain	1	6.0	165
yeast	1	11.3	175
Dried Beef	2 oz. (approx. 10 slices)	2.2	115
creamed	1/2 cup	3.0	190
Duck			
domestic roasted meat only	4 oz.	28.4	355
Eggs			
hard or soft cooked	1 large	6.0	80
scrambled	1 large	8.0	110
Eggnog, 8% fat	1/2 cup	9.5	186
Figs	1 large	.5	60
Fig bars	2 bars	2.0	100
Fish Sticks breaded	2 sticks (3-3/4"x1" x1/2")	4.0	80
Frankfurter	1	15.0	170
Fruit cocktail			
canned in heavy syrup	1/2 cup	.5	97
Fruit drinks			
Apricot nectar	1/2 cup	.1	70
Cranberry juice	1/2 cup	.1	80
Grape drink	1/2 cup	.0	70
Grape juice	1/2 cup	.0	85
Grapefruit juice, unsweetened	1/2 cup	.2	50
Grapefruit juice, sweetened	1/2 cup	.2	65
Lemonade	1/2 cup	.0	70
Orange-apricot	1/2 cup	.2	60
Peach nectar	1/2 cup	.1	60
Pear nectar	1/2 cup	.0	65
Pineapple-grapefruit	1/2 cup	.1	170
Pineapple-orange	1/2 cup	.0	70
Gelatin dessert			
all flavors prepared (Jell-O)	1/2 cup	.0	81
plain	1/2 cup	.0	70
fruit added	f1/2 cup	.0	80
Goose, roasted, meat only	4 oz.	21.0	266
Gooseberries, fresh	1/2 pound	1.0	88
Grapes, raw (American type)	1/2 cup	.5	45
Grapefruit			
pink or red	1/2 grapefruit	.4	50
white	1/2 grapefruit	.4	45
Gravy	2 tbsp.	3.2	35
Grouper, raw, flesh only	4 ozx.	1.2	99
Gum chewing			
Beechnut	1 stick	.0	10
Doublemint, Juicy Fruit, Spearmint	1 stick	.0	8
Gumdrops	1 oz.	.2	100
Haddock			
breaded, fried	3 oz.	5.0	140
frozen, fillets	4 oz. 2 fillets	.8	88
Halibut, fresh or frozen, broiled with 2 tsp. butter	4 oz.	10.9	188
Ham			
lean & fat	3 oz.	18.0	245
cured (lean)	3 oz.	4.6	160
Hamburger			
regular	3 oz.	19.6	245
lean	3 oz.	12.2	185
Hard Candy	1 oz.	.3	110
Herring			
raw, Atlantic	4 oz.	10.4	200
pickled	4 oz.	12.7	253
smoked, hard	4 oz.	13.0	340
Hickorynuts shelled	1/4 pound	73.2	767
Honey	1 tbsp.	.0	65
Honeydew Melon	1 wedge	.4	50
Ice Cream			
regular	1/2 cup	7.0	130
softserve	1/2 cup	10.0	165
chocolate	1/2 pt.	11.5	191
strawberry	1/2 pt.	10.3	174
vanilla	1/2 pt.	9.4	176
French chocolate	1/2 pt.	14.9	250
French vanilla	1/2 pt.	14.9	247
bar chocolate coating	3 oz.	11.5	162
sandwich	1	11.0	208
cane, sugar	1	.3	37
cone, waffle	1	.0	19
Ice milk			
hardened	1/2 cup	3.5	100
soft serve	1/2 cup	4.6	135
Jam and preserves	1 tbsp.	.0	55
Jelly	1 tbsp.	.0	50
Jelly beans	1 tbsp.	.1	105
Kidney beef, braised	4 oz.	4.0	287
Kingfish, raw flesh only	4 oz.	3.9	119
Knockwurst	4 oz.	27.9	317
Lamb			
chops, lean & fat	3 oz.	25.0	300
chops, lean only	3 oz.	8.0	160
leg roast, lean & fat	3 oz.	23.0	285
leg roast, lean only	3 oz.	7.0	160
shoulder roast, lean & fat	3 oz.	23.0	285
shoulder roast, lean only	3 oz.	8.0	175
Lemon juice	1 tbsp.	.0	5
Lemonade			
frozen, concentrated	1/2 cup	.3	55
frozen, diluted	8 oz. glass	.4	109
Lettuce			
iceberg	1/2 cup, shredded	.5	5
	1/2 pound	1.0	28
romaine	1/2 pound	1.0	26
Limeade, frozen, diluted	8 oz. glass	.4	102
Liver			
beef, fried	2 oz.	6.0	130
	4 oz.	12.0	260
chicken, simmered	4 oz.	6.2	187
Liver paste, see Pate de foie gras			
Liverwurst, fresh	4 oz.	31.0	350
Lobster, canned or cooked, meat only	4 oz.	1.1	108
Loganberries, fresh	1/2 cup	.0	45
Macaroni, boiled 14-20 min. drained	1/2 cup	.3	78
Mackerel, fresh or frozen, broiled with 2 tsp. butter	4 oz.	20.1	262
	3 oz.	15.1	200

Food	Amount	Grams of Fat	Calories
Mangos, fresh	1 average, 3 1/4" long	.6	134
Marshmallows	1 oz.	.0	90
Milk			
Buttermilk	1 cup	2.4	90
Skim	1 cup	.4	90
2%	1 cup	5.0	145
Whole	1 cup	9.0	160
Evaporated	1/2 cup	10.0	175
Condensed	1/2 cup	14.0	490
Chocolate	1 cup	12.0	240
Chocolate drink mix (water added)	1 cup	3.0	190
Chocolate drink mix (milk added)	1 cup	9.1	215
Malted	1 cup	10.0	245
Shake	12 oz.	28.0	515
Goats whole	8 oz.	10.1	163
Molasses			
blackstrap (dark)	1 tbsp.	.0	45
cane (light)	1 tbsp.	.0	50
Muffins			
corn	1 muffin	4.2	125
bran	1 muffin	5.1	105
blueberry	1 muffin	4.3	110
Mushrooms	1/2 cup	.2	20
Mustard greens	1/2 cup	.5	15
Nectarines, fresh	1 average	.5	30
Noodles, enriched	3/4 cup	1.8	150
Nuts			
almond (shelled)	2 tbsp.	9.8	105
Brazil nuts (shelled)	2 tbsp.	12.2	115
cashew nuts	2 tbsp.	9.7	100
coconut, shredded	2 tbsp.	4.5	55
macadamia	6 nuts	10.5	104
peanuts, roasted	2 tbsp.	9.7	105
peanut butter	2 tbsp.	15.7	95
pecans (shelled)	2 tbsp.	12.5	95
walnuts	2 tbsp.	11.5	100
Oats, Oatmeal, see Cereals			
Oil			
corn	1 tbsp.	14.0	120
cottonseed, winterized	1 tbsp.	14.0	128
olive	1 tbsp.	14.0	125
peanut	1 tbsp.	14.0	124
safflower	1 tbsp.	14.0	128
salad or cooking	1tbsp.	14.0	124
soybean	1 tbsp.	14.0	125
Okra, cooked	1/2 cup, sliced	.2	25
Olives			
green	3 large	2.0	15
ripe	2 large	2.0	15
Onions, raw	1/2 cup	.4	35
Orange	1 orange (2. 5/8" dia.)	.5	55
dehydrated crystals	1/2 cup	.5	58
Oysters, raw	1/2 cup	2.0	80
Pancakes			
plain or buttermilk	3-1/2 cakes, (4" across)	10.3	210
wheat	1 cake	4.0	60
buck wheat	1 cake	4.0	55
Papayas, fresh	1/2 pound	.5	60
Parsnips, cooked	1/2 cup	.2	50
Pate de foie gras, canned	1 oz.	12.4	131
Peach			
fresh	1 medium	.3	40
canned, water packed	1/2 cup	.2	40
canned, heavy syrup	1/2 cup	.4	100
dried, unsweetened	1/2 cup	.5	100
Peanut Brittle	1 oz.	2.9	120
Pears			
canned, water packed	1/2 cup	.5	40
canned, heavy syrup	1/2 cup	.5	95
raw	1 pear	1.0	100
Peas			
blackeyed, dry, cooked	1/2 cup	.5	95
green, canned	1/2 cup	.5	65
split, dry, cooked	1/2 cup	.5	145
Pecans, shelled	1/4 pound	77.0	779
Peppers			
green, raw	1/4 pod	.0	4
sweet, green, raw, seeded	1 average	.2	14
green, cooked	1 medium	.2	15
holt, red, chili powder	1 tbsp.	2.0	50
Perch			
ocean, breaded & fried	3 oz.	10.4	195
fresh or frozen, baked with 2 tsp. butter	4 oz.	12.8	160
Pickle relish			
sour	1 tbsp.	.0	2
sweet	1 tbsp.	.2	18
Pickles, dill, medium	1 pickle, 3-1/4" long	.1	15
Pie			
apple, 2 crust	1/7 or 9" dia. pie (of 1 sector 4")	12.0	300
blueberry, 2 crust	1/7 of 9" dia. pie of 1 sector 4"	13.0	285
cherry, 2 crust	1 sector	13.0	350
chocolate meringue	1 sector	15.0	285
coconut custard	1 sector	14.3	270
custard, 1 crust	1 sector	13.0	250
lemon meringue	f1 sector	13.5	270
mince	1 sector	14.0	320
peach	1 sector	14.0	430
pecan	1 sector	19.0	430
pumpkin, 1 crust	1 sector	13.0	275
raisin	1 sector	13.0	320
rhubarb	1 sector	13.0	300
strawberry	1 sector	7.0	185
Pig's feet, pickled	4 oz.	18.3	226
Pike, raw, blue, flesh only	4 oz.	1.2	102
Pimientos, canned	1 averaged	.0	10
Pineapple			
fresh	1/2 cup	.4	40
canned, crushed, heavy syrup	1/2 cup	.5	95
sliced, canned	1 slice	.5	80
Pineapple juice, canned, unsweetened	1/2 cup	.4	70
Pistachia nuts, shelled	1/4 pound	60.0	674
Pizza, with cheese, no meat	1 section, 5-1/2"	10.0	
	or 1/8 of 14"	10.0	185
	dia. pie 5" section	9.0	155
Plums			
fresh	5 plums	.3	35
canned	1/2 cup	.7	105
Pomegranates, fresh	1/2 pound	.4	80
Popcorn	1 cup	2.0	40
Pork & beans	1/2 cup	3.5	155
Pork chops			
lean & fat (1 chop)	(2.3 oz.)	21.0	300
lean only (1 chop)	(2 oz.)	7.0	150
Pork roast, lean & fat	3 oz.	24.0	310
Pork sausage, link	4 links or 4 oz.	22.0	250
Potato			
without skin, boiled	1 medium	.8	145
baked	1 medium	.5	90
chips	10 chips	8.0	115
french fries in oil	10 pc.	7.0	200
frozen, oven heated	10 pc.	5.0	170

Food	Amount	Grams of Fat	Calories
Potatoes (*continued*)			
mashed with milk	3/4 cup (1 potato mashed)	1.0	95
hash browned	1/2 cup	9.0	175
au gratin	1/2 cup	9.3	180
scalloped without cheese	1/2 cup	4.5	125
Potato salad			
with mayonnaise	1/2 cup	9.0	180
with salad dressing	1/2 cup	2.0	125
Pretzels			
twist	1 pretzel	.6	60
stick	5 regular	.1	10
Prunes, fresh or canned, unsweetened	1/2 cup	.5	125
Prune juice	1/2 cup	.2	100
Puddings and pie filings, mix, prepared as directed			
all flavors except lemon	1/2 cup	3.7	168
banana	1/2 cup	4.3	165
butterscotch	1/2 cup	4.8	190
chocolate	1/2 cup	4.8	190
chocolate, Dark 'N Sweet	1/2 cup	4.9	195
custard	1/2 cup	5.4	145
lemon	1/2 cup	3.8	125
lemon chiffon filling	1/2 cup	4.0	144
tapioca, chocolate	1/2 cup	7.4	185
tapioca, vanilla	1/2 cup	6.4	170
vanilla	1/2 cup	4.3	165
Puddings, "instant" mix, prepared as directed			
all flavors	1/2 cup	4.4	185
banana cream	1/2 cup	4.3	175
butterscotch	1/2 cup	4.3	175
caramel nut	1/2 cup	4.9	195
chocolate	1/2 cup	5.0	200
lemon	1/2 cup	4.3	180
mocha nut	1/2 cup	5.0	200
vanilla	1/2 cup	4.3	40
Pumpkin, canned	1/2 cup	.5	40
Quail, raw, boned	4 oz.	5.1	172
Rabbit, domestic, meat only, stewed	4 oz.	12.0	246
Radishes, raw	5 medium	.0	5
Raisins, seedless	1/2 cup	.0	240
Raspberries, red, frozen	1/2 cup	.5	120
Rhubarb, cooke,d sugar added	1/2 cup	.3	190
Rib Roast			
lean & fat	3 oz.	30.0	375
lean only	3 oz.	14.0	205
Rice			
brown, cooked	1/2 cup	.6	100
white, precooked, cooked	1/2 cup	.1	105
Rice-A-Roni			
beef	1/2 cup	7.3	160
chicken	1/2 cup	7.2	157
wild	1/2 cup	4.1	141
Round Road			
lean & fat	3 oz.	13.0	220
lean only	3 oz.	5.5	160
Salad dressings & fats			
French	1 tbsp.	6.0	65
Blue Cheese	1 tbsp.	8.0	75
Italian	1 tbsp.	7.1	85
Mayonnaise	1 tbsp.	4.9	100
Russian	1 tbsp.	7.8	75
Thousand Island	1 tbsp.	8.0	80
vegetable	1 tbsp.	14.0	110
lard	1 tbsp.	12.8	115
salad or cooking oil	1 tbsp.	6.0	65
Low calorie dressing			
French	1 tbsp.	.4	15
Italian	1 tbsp.	.4	10
Thousand Island	1 tbsp.	.8	25

Food	Amount	Grams of Fat	Calories
Salami	2 oz.	17.0	175
Salmon, pink, canned, including bones	3 oz. or about 1/2 cup	5.0	120
Sandwich spread relish	1 tbsp.	2.8	57
Sardines	3 oz.	9.0	175
Sauces			
white , made with butter or margarine	1/2 cup	15.0	202
barbecue	1 tbsp.	.3	14
chili	1 tbsp.	.0	15
cheese	1/2 cup	16.0	205
Sauerkraut, canned, solids & liquid	1/2 cup	.2	20
Scallops, breaded, fried, frozen, reheated	4 oz.	13.6	220
Sherbet	1/2 cup	2.7	152
Shortening	1 tbsp.	11.0	103
Shrimp	3 oz.	1.3	100
Soft drinks			
cola (Coca-Cola)	8 oz. glass	.0	96
cream soda	8 oz. glass	.0	105
ginger ale	8 oz. glass	.0	85
ginger beer (Schweppes)	8 oz. glass	.0	96
Kook-Aid, all flavor, prepared with water	8 oz. glass	.0	91
Mountain Dew	8 oz. glass	.0	116
quinine water (Schweppes)	8 oz. glass	.0	88
root beer	8 oz. glass	.0	96
Seven-up	8 oz. glass	.0	97
Sprite	8 oz. glass	.0	96
Wink	8 oz. glass	.0	119
Sole, fillets, frozen (Birds Eye)	2 fillets , 4 oz.	.8	88
Soup, canned, condensed, diluted with equal amount water			
bean with pork	1 cup	6.0	170
beef noodle	1 cup	3.0	65
bouillon broth	1 cup	.0	30
chicken gumbo	1 cup	1.4	55
chicken noodle	1 cup	2.0	60
chicken vegetable	1 cup	2.8	74
chicken with rice	1 cup	1.9	50
clam chowder, Manhattan	1 cup	3.0	80
cream of asparagus with water	1 cup	4.1	65
cream of asparagus with milk	1 cup	8.2	180
cream of chicken	1 cup	10.0	180
cream of mushroom with water	1 cup	10.0	135
cream of mushroom with milk	1 cup	14.0	215
green pea	1 cup	2.9	130
minestrone	1 cup	3.0	105
onion	1 cup	1.7	45
oyster stew with water	1 cup	8.0	120
oyster stew with milk	1 cup	12.0	200
split pea	1 cup	3.0	146
tomato with water	1 cup	3.0	90
tomato with milk	1 cup	7.0	170
turkey noodle	1 cup	2.0	81
vegetable with beef broth	1 cup	2.0	80
vegetarian vegetable	1 cup	2.0	77
Spaghetti, cooked	3/4 cup	.6	115
Spaghetti with meatballs	3/4 cup	9.0	250
Spaghetti with tomato sauce & cheese	3/4 cup	2.5	195
Spaghetti with meat balls & tomato sauce	1 cup	12.0	330
Spinach, canned, drained	1/2 cup	.5	25
Squash			
hard winter, baked, mashed	1/2 cup	.5	65
light summer, cooked	1/2 cup, diced	.1	15
Steak, broiled			
Sirloin, lean and fat	3 oz.	20.5	330

Food	Amount	Grams of Fat	Calories
Sirloin, lean only	3 oz.	9.9	175
Round, lean & fat	3 oz.	9.8	220
Round, lean only	3 oz.	6.0	160
Strawberries			
fresh	1/2 cup	.1	30
frozen	1/2 cup or (1/2 of 10 oz. carton)	.5	140
Sugar			
brown	1 tbsp.	.0	51
white	1 tbsp.	.0	40
Sweet potatoes			
baked	1 medium	1.0	155
candied	1 medium	6.0	295
canned	1/2 cup	.8	140
Syrup			
chocolate, thin type	1 tbsp.	.1	45
chocolate, fudge type	1 tbsp.	.2	60
corn, light or dark	1 tbsp.	.0	60
Tangerine, fresh	1 medium	.2	40
Tea	1 cup	.0	4
Tomatoe juice, canned	1/2 cup	.2	25
Tomato catsup	1 tbsp.	.1	15
Tomatoes			
canned, solids & liquid	1/2 cup	.5	25
fresh	1 medium	.6	40
Tongue, beef	3 oz.	17.0	210
pickled	4 oz.	21.0	303
Toppings, Ice cream and dessert			
black raspberry	1 tbsp.	.0	40
butterscotch	1 tbsp.	.5	52
caramel	1 tbsp.	1.4	72
cherry	1 tbsp.	.0	40
chocolate fudge	1 tbsp.	2.6	66
chocolate mint (Hershey)	1 tbsp.	.4	61
Dream Whip, prepared	1 tbsp.	.4	14
marshmallow creme	1 tbsp.	.0	45
pineapple	1 tbsp.	.0	40
strawberry	1 tbsp.	.0	40
vanilla caramel	1 tbsp.	1.5	80
whipped, pressurized	1 tbsp.	.9	10
Trout, rainbow, canned	4 oz.	4.9	237
Tuna, canned in oil	3 oz. or 1/2 cup	7.0	170
Turkey			
roasted, light meat	3 oz.	2.8	150
roasted , dark meat	3 oz.	4.3	175
Turnip green, cooked	1/2 cup	.1	15
Turnips, cooked	1/2 cup, diced	.2	20
Vienna sausages	3 sausages	12.0	120
Waffles			
frozen (Aunt Jemima	1 dbl. waffle	4.3	128
made with milk & egg	1 waffle, 7" dia.	12.0	205
Water chestnuts, Chinese, raw	1/2 pound	.2	136
Watercress, raw	10 sprigs	.0	5
Watermelon	1 wedge, 4"x8"	1.0	110
Weiners	1	16.3	170
Yogurt			
skimmed milk	1 cup	.4	125
whole milk	1 cup	8.0	240

Common Fast Foods

Food	Amount	Grams of Fat	Calories
Hamburger			
Burger Chef	3 oz.	13.0	258
Burger King, Whopper	9 oz.	32.0	663
McDonald's	7-1/2 oz.	31.0	590
Big Mac		9.0	249
Single		18.0	353
Double		21.0	415
Quarter Pounder		42.0	826
Half Pounder		80.0	
Wendy's, Old Fashion Single	6-1/2 oz.	22.0	415
Jack-in-the-Box, Jumbo Jack	8-1/4 oz.	34.0	535
Cheeseburger Meal			
(add 107 calories for cheese) Quarter Pounder, large fries, 8 oz. cola, cherry turnover		64.6	1,090
Chicken			
Kentucky Fried Chicken			
Snack Box	6-3/4 oz.	22.0	408
Original Recipe dinner	3 pieces	46.0	830
Extra Crisp dinner	3 pieces	54.0	950
Drumstick	1 piece	11.0	221
Family Bucket	15 pieces	156.0	3,300
Meal, (3 pieces of chicken, coleslaw, mashed potatoes, gravy, biscuit, 8 oz. cola)		75.0	1,088
Fish			
Burger King, Whaler	7 oz.	27.0	585
Long John Silver's			
Fish sandwich	1 fillet	31.0	345
Fish dinner	2 pieces	38.0	483
Fish only	1 piece	11.0	170
Coleslaw	1 serving	8.0	122
McDonald's Fish Sandwich	4-1/2 oz.	25.7	385
Sandwiches			
Hardee's Roast Beef	4-1/2 oz.	9.0	350
Diary Queen			
Hot Dog	regular	15.0	265
Chili Dog	regular	20.0	335
Cheese Dog	regular	19.0	330
A &W			
Foot Long Hot Dog		33.0	500
Foot Long Chili Dog		40.0	575
Roast Beef Sandwich meal, (french fries, 8 oz. cola)		28.0	655
Side Orders & Specialties			
French fries	regular	11.0	196
French fries	large	18.0	275
Onion rings		16.0	300
Egg McMuffin	1	14.0	352
Wendy's chili	10 oz.	5.0	265
Thin & Crispy Cheese Pizza	1/2 of 10" pie	16.0	455
Thin & Crispy Pepperoni Pizza	1/2 of 10" pie	24.0	565
Apple Turnover		14.3	295
Cherry Turnover		13.6	3k02
Taco Bell			
Taco	1	8.0	186
Bean Burrito	1	12.0	325
Encherito		21.0	420
Fried Beans		5.0	174
tostada	1	6.0	185

Fast Food Restaurant

Food	Amount	Grams of Fat	Calories
Arby's			
Beef & Cheese Sandwich		24.0	450
Beef & Cheddar		26.8	484
Roast Beef Sandwich		15.0	350
Junior Roast Beef Sandwich		9.0	220
Super Roast Beef Sandwich		22.1	620
Roast Beef Deluxe		20.0	486
French Dip		15.0	366
Club Sandwich		30.0	560
Ham 'n Cheese Sandwich		17.0	380
Chicken Breast Sandwich		25.0	584
Turkey Deluxe Sandwich		24.0	510
Turkey Sandwich		16.6	410
Potato Cake		4.0	80
French Fries, Small		13.6	216
French Fries, Large		21.6	343
Arby's Sauce, 1 pkg.		.0	10
Horsey Sauce, 1 pkg.		5.0	45
Apple Turnover		14.0	310
Cherry Turnover		13.0	320
Blueberry Turnover		13.2	340

Food	Grams of Fat	Calories
Burger King		
Hamburger	25.0	290
Whopper	27.0	630
with cheese	35.0	740
Whopper Junior	20.1	370
with cheese	27.0	420
Double Beef Whopper	52.0	850
with cheese	60.0	950
Cheeseburger	17.0	350
Double Cheeseburger	32.0	530
Bacon Double Cheeseburger	31.0	600
Beef Sandwich	26.0	64.4
Chicken Sandwich	40.0	620
Fish Sandwich	38.0	646
Ham & Cheese Sandwich	24.0	573
French Fries	11.0	210
Onion Rings	16.0	270
Shake	12.0	340
Apple Pie	12.0	340
Vanilla Shake	11.0	340
Specialty Ham/Cheese Sandwich	32.0	550
Speciality Chicken Sandwich	38.0	690
Whaler Sandwich w/cheese	36.0	590
Whaler Sandwich	27.0	540
Dairy Queen		
Banana Split	15.0	540
Big Brazier		
Deluxe	24.0	470
Regular	23.0	457
with Cheese	30.0	553
Brazier Cheese Dog	19.0	330
Brazier Chili Dog	20.0	330
Brazier Dog	15.0	273
Brazier French Fries		
Large	16.0	320
Small	10.0	200
Brazier Onion Rings	17.0	300
Brazier Regular	9.0	260
Brazier with Cheese	14.0	318
Buster Bar	22.0	390
Cone:		
Large	10.0	340
Regular	7.0	230
Small	3.0	110
Dipped Cone:		
Large	20.0	450
Regular	13.0	300
Small	7.0	150
DQ Float	8.0	330
DQ Freeze	13.0	520
DQ Parfait	11.0	460
DQ Sandwich	4.0	140
Dilly Bar	15.0	240
Fiesta Sundae	22.0	570
Malt or Shake:		
Large	28.0	840
Regular	20.0	600
Small	11.0	340
Mr. Misty:		
Float	.0	440
Freeze	.0	500
Kiss	.0	70
Sundae:		
Large	9.0	400
Regular	7.0	290
Small	4.0	170
Super Brazier	48.0	783
Chili Dog	33.0	555
Dog	30.0	518
Dog with cheese	36.0	593
Dunkin' Donuts		
Cake and Chocolate Cake Donuts		240
Fancies (Coffee Rolls, Danish, etc.)*	14.0-22.0	215
Munchkins**	10.0-15.0	
Cake and Chocolate Cake Yeast Raised		66
Yeast Raised Donuts***		160

*Add 40-50 cal. for filling & topping
**Add 10-15 cal. for filling & topping
***Add 5-10 cal. per donut for glaze

Kentucky Fried Chicken

	Grams of Fat Original		Grams of Fat Extra Crispy	
Breast	11.7	199	17.8	286
Drumstick	6.5	117	9.0	155
Keel	18.0	236	23.0	297
Rib	13.0	241	18.0	
Thigh	17.5	257	23.4	343
Wing	9.0	146	13.5	210
9 Pice Dinner	120.0	1,892	240.0	
Chicken Dinner*	30.0	830	55.0	950
Chicken Breast Sandwich	22.5	620	45.0	436
Kentucky Fries	6.7			184
Mashed Potatoes	.9			64
Gravy	1.8			23
Coleslaw	7.5			122
Rolls	1.1			61
Corn	2.8			169

*Dinner—Mashed potatoes & gravy, coleslaw, roll, and 3 pieces of chicken.

Food	Grams of Fat	Calories
Hardee's		
Hamburger	10.0	305
Cheeseburger	14.0	335
Big Cheese	29.0	495
Big Deluxe	30.0	546
Big Roast Beef	11.0	418
Big Twin	25.0	447
Ham and Cheese	12.0	376
Roast Beef Sandwich	9.0	376
Hot Dog	17.0	346
French Fries:		
Large	17.0	381
Small	11.0	239
Chicken Fillet	13.0	510
Ham Biscuit w/Egg	19.0	349
Egg (medium)	8.0	108
Jelly	.0	49
Steak Biscuit w/Egg	32.0	419
Milkshake	9.0	391
Apple Turnover	12.0	281
Long John Silver's		
Breaded Clams	34.0	617
Breaded Oysters	19.0	441
Carbonated Drinks (10 oz).	.0	120
Chicken Plansk (4 pieces)	23.0	457
with fries	39.0	745
Clam Chowder (8 oz.)	3.0	107
Clam Dinner	50.0	891
Coleslaw	8.0	138
Corn on the Cob	4.0	176
Dit Carbonated Drinks	.0	10
Fish and Chicken Dinner	49.0	837
Fish/Fryes	49.0	837
Fish/More	55.0	894
Fish Sandwich	31.0	337
French Fries	16.0	288
Fish with Batter		
3 pieces	22.0	366
3 pieces	33.0	549
Hush Puppies	7.0	153

Food	Grams of Fat	Calories
Milk—8 oz.	5.0	159
Ocean Scallops	13.0	283
Oyster Dinner	36.0	867
Peg Legs w/Batter	28.0	350
with Fries	44.0	725
Scallop Dinner	28.0	709
Seafood Platter	35.0	894
Shrimp w/Batter	13.0	268
Treasurer Chest	33.0	506
McDonald's		
Big Mac	35.7	563
Cheeseburger	14.1	307
Cones:		
Cake	5.2	185
Sugar	4.5	170
Cookies:		
Chocolaty Chips	16.3	342
McDonaldland	10.8	308
Chicken McNuggets (6)	19.0	310
Sauces for McNuggests:		
Honey	0.0	50
Hot Mustard	2.1	63
Barbeque	.4	60
Sweet & Sour	.3	64
Egg McMuffin	11.2	290
English Muffin	5.3	187
Filet-of-Fish	25.0	432
French FRies	11.5	220
Hamburger	9.8	220
Hash Browns	7.0	125
Hotcakes w/Butter/Syrup	10.3	500
Pie:		
Apple	14.3	253
Cherry	13.6	260
Quarter Pounder	21.7	424
with cheese	30.7	524
Sausage	18.6	
Scrambled Eggs	13.0	
Shakes:		
Chocolate	9.0	383
Strawberry	8.7	362
Vanilla	8.4	352
Sundaes:		
Caramel	10.0	328
Hot Fudge	10.8	310
Strawberry	8.7	289
Biscuits	12.0	260
Sausage Biscuit	18.0	582
Biscuit w/Bacon, Egg & Cheese	26.4	440

Pizza Hut

	Grams of Fat	Thin/ Crispy	Thick/ Chewy
Standard:			
Cheese	5.4	180	208
Pepperoni	11.5	202	224
Pork/Mushroom	6.2	196	227
Super Supreme	18.0	266	300
Superstyle:			
Cheese	8.6	213	235
Pepperoni	11.5	233	244
Prik/Mushroom	11.0	230	244
Supreme	15.0	216	244

Values for 1/8 slice of medium pizza.

Food	Grams of Fat	Calories
Red Lobster		
Breaded Fried Pollock or Whiting	1.0	175-200
Catfish, Fresh Water	10.0	788-117
Chicken, Skinless-4 pcs.	12.0	452
Clams	21.0	89
Cod	1.0	79-97
Crab, Snow	2.0	93
Egg	6.0	163
Flounder	1.0	84-90
Garlic Bread, 1 slice	2.0	13
Grouper	1.0	83-94
Haddock	1.0	79
Halibut	1.0	77
Hamburger Pattie	28.0	268
Hush Puppies, 2	12.0	206
Lobster	3.0	95
Oysters	4.0	54-92
Perch	4.0	88
Pollock	1.0	86-94
Potato	1.0	76
Scallops	2.0	87
Shrimp	2.0	88-97
Sirloin Steak	15.0	353
Snapper	1.0	100-105
Sole	1.0	80-85
Tuna	6.0	122-126
Whiting	2.0	105
Broiled Fisherman's Platter		992
(lobster, sea bass, scallop, deviled crab, hush puppies, coleslaw, and baked potato)		36.0
Broiled Stuff Flounder		1028
(fillets stuffed with crab meat filling, hush puppies, coleslaw, and baked potato)	31.0	
Mariner's Platter		944
(fried shrimp, fish fillet, oysters, fish fingers, deviled crab cake, fried fish fillet, hush puppies, coleslaw, and baked potato)	61.0	
Sampler Platter		808
(broiled lobster, broiled Alaskan split crab legs, fried shrimp, hush puppies, coleslaw and baked potato)	32.0	
Shore Platter		832
(fried shrimp, scallops, oysters, fish fillet, hush puppies, coleslaw, and baked potato)	34.0	
Steak and Lobster		1540
(sirloin stake, broiled rock lobster tail, hush puppies, coleslaw and baked potato)	74.0	
Taco Bell		
Bean Burrito	10.8	343
Beef Burrito	21.0	466
Beefy Tostado	15.0	291
Bellbeefer	7.0	221
Bellbeefer w/cheese	12.0	278
Burrito Supreme	16.0	404
Enchirito	16.9	454
Pintos 'n cheese	6.0	168
Taco	8.6	186
Tostada	6.0	179
Taco Salad	6.0	179
Taco Salad	64.0	941
Wendy's		
Cheeseburger:		
Single cheese	34.0	580
Double cheese	48.0	800
Triple cheese	68.0	1040
Chili	8.0	230
French Fries	16.0	330
Frosty	16.0	390
Hamburger:		
Single	26.0	470
Double	40.0	670
Chicken Sandwich	30.0	463
Chicken w/cheese	35.0	496
Taco Salad	64.0	460
1 oz. serving:		
Alfalfa Sprouts	.0	10
American Cheese	7.0	70

Food	Grams of Fat	Calories
Wendy's *(continued)*		
Bacon Bits	.0	80
Bean Sprouts	.0	10
Beets	.0	10
Bell Peppers	.0	6
Breadsticks	7.0	240
Broccoli	.0	10
Carrots	.0	12
Cauliflower	.0	8
Cheddar Cheese	6.0	90
Chow Mein Noodles	9.0	160
Coleslaw	5.0	45
Cottage Cheese	1.0	30
Croutons	6.0	120

Food	Amount	Grams of Fat	Calories
Cucumbers		.0	4
Eggs		2.0	45
Garbanzo Beans		.0	25
Gelatin Parfailt		2.0	30
Green Peas		.0	20
Kidney Beans		.0	25
Lettuce, Iceberg		.0	4
Lettuce, Romaine		.0	6
Mild Green Pepperoncini		.0	8
Mushrooms		.0	10
Parmesan Cheese		9.0	140
Pineapple Chunks		.0	18
Sunflower Seeds & Raisins		10.0	140
Tomatoes		.0	6